"I've known Ethan Brown for a long time. But only after reading his book, did I really understand who he is and the challenges he's facing. Ethan is a wonderful young man, and his willingness to share his struggles through this book should be a blessing to everyone who reads it."

—**Dan Scott,**
host of the Dan Scott Show,
play-by-play voice for the Greenville
Drive baseball team

"I lived 25 years of my life without knowing of neurofibromatosis and its impact on individuals and families. Thanks to Ian Desmond, I'm not only aware of the disease but I also have the privilege of calling fighters in the NF community my friends. Among those is Ethan Brown, who embodies all that is good in this world: kindness, humor, and an uncanny ability to positively impact all those he meets. His story is one that transforms lives. I know this because I'm a testimony of it! Thank you, Ethan, for being vulnerable enough to share your story and impact so many."

—**Taylor McGregor,**
ESPN college football reporter,
field reporter for the Chicago Cubs

"Ethan's story is a reminder that we cannot go through life on our own. The power of prayer, family, and friendship help us endure the trials along the way. I'm blessed that God put Ethan in my life and gave me the opportunity to read this book. What a testimony of faith and perseverance."

—D. J. Johnson,
former Colorado Rockies pitcher,
player for the Tohoku Rakuten Golden Eagles
of the Nippon Professional Baseball Organization

"I truly enjoyed the journey and being part of the struggle that you are still fighting today. Reading this book brought back some great memories over the last 10+ years. We need to be reminded, and you have done so with this book! I am sure others who read this will see the similarities with their lives and their struggles. I hate this struggle for you, but you have done a heck of a job dealing with the hand you have been dealt and that is why you will always be 'my hero'!"

—Sam Kelly,
former owner/boss at Sam Group, Lubbock, Texas

THE FIGHT OF MY LIFE

Persevering through Neurofibromatosis

ETHAN W. BROWN

LUCIDBOOKS

The Fight of My Life
Persevering through Neurofibromatosis

Published by Lucid Books in Houston, TX
www.LucidBooksPublishing.com

ISBN: 978-1-63296-426-7
eISBN: 978-1-63296-427-4

Special Sales: Most Lucid Books titles are available in special quantity discounts. Custom imprinting or excerpting can also be done to fit special needs. For standard bulk orders, go to www.lucidbooksbulk.com. For specialty press or large orders, contact Lucid Books at books@lucidbookspublishing.com.

TABLE OF CONTENTS

*This book is dedicated to my family—
especially my parents.
They have been on this journey with me for over
10 years. We haven't always seen eye to eye, but I
wouldn't be here today if not for y'all. I wanted this
book to be in print for Mom's birthday but couldn't
finish by July—so consider it a belated gift.*

*It's also for all the NF fighters out there. I was placed
here for a reason. I don't want to be like the servant
Jesus speaks of in Matthew 25 who was given one
talent and did nothing with it. I want to be like the
other two and hear, "Well done."*

Ethan

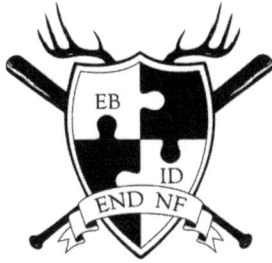

FOREWORD

Ethan and I met around 2011 or 2012 on Twitter (believe it or not). I was a young Major League Baseball player trying to find my way, and my agent suggested I start a social media account to capitalize on some of the financial benefits. I was reluctant at first, so he offered to hire a company to run it for me. They set up my profile and did their best to speak on my behalf, but it didn't take long for me to realize this wasn't going to work and that nobody could pretend to be me. I took the account over not long after that and started following people, specifically in this case, a Christian athletes outreach feed. Ethan had posted to them asking for prayer. We didn't know each other; he was a Braves fan and I played for their rival, the Nationals, at the time. I had never done anything like this before, but I decided to message him back. "Hey man, I'll pray for you," I said. That message turned out to be the first notch on the wall, and we've been notching away ever since.

Soon after we connected, Ethan and I got to meet when he and his family drove to one of my games at Turner Field. After the game, I left them passes to go down to the tunnel—I was always the last one out, so they were the last people in the tunnel. I'm not sure how thrilled they were about that, but nonetheless, they waited. At this time, Ethan could walk, talk, hear, and had full motor function. I had arranged to get him a signed Chipper Jones ball, so I gave the ball to him, and we chatted for a bit. Then, Ethan did something that probably etched our friendship in stone forever when he offered his hand and asked me to feel a tumor on it. As I carefully touched it, Ethan, being the sass that he is, went into a full convulsion, sending me jumping back in a full panic. I'd never touched a tumor before and had no idea what to expect. He was joking, of course—something I most certainly would have done if I were in his shoes. We laugh about that moment to this day.

Ethan's sense of humor is one thing that always sticks out to me. While it's maybe not as good as he thinks it is, it's pretty good, and we can go back and forth with each other like brothers. If you were to look at the hundreds of thousands of texts we've sent each other over the years, you'd never know I was a Major League Baseball player or that Ethan has a genetic disorder stealing his physical body. We just are who we are to each other, and it's pretty much the definition of unconditional love. It's no doubt that we make each other mad, but it never lasts long. We have each other's backs.

Many times when I have been emotionally or physically drained, I think about all that Ethan and the other kids I've met over the years with NF have endured. And I realize that *I can do it*—I can face my challenges. At times I have walked to the plate in some of my biggest moments at bat thinking of Ethan and all the kids like him and saying to myself, "This is nothing compared to the fight they are going through." This focus has always brought the calm I needed in the moment.

The NF community embodies their slogan: "I Know a Fighter." I don't believe I have ever met a person with NF who had a "poor me" attitude. NF may be a genetic disorder, but I'm almost certain there is a positive genetic effect that gives these kids an infinite amount of resolve. It's a gene I don't have in me on my own, but over the years, they have passed it on to me.

I couldn't be prouder of Ethan and his resolve. He and his family have been through so much, yet he continues to push on and inspire people like me every day. He's done things in his life that most people can only dream about. He's rallied people together and figuratively and literally talked people off the edge. He's a loyal supporter and advocate, a great friend, and a brother. I'm so proud to sit here writing this foreword, knowing soon I'll be able to call him an *author*. Ethan Brown, I couldn't be prouder of you, brother. You've done it! Your legacy will live on forever through this book, and it's because of your hard work and determination. Congratulations, my friend. I love you.

Your Friend,
Ian Desmond, Major League Baseball player,
Colorado Rockies, Two-time All-Star, Washington
Nationals and Texas Rangers

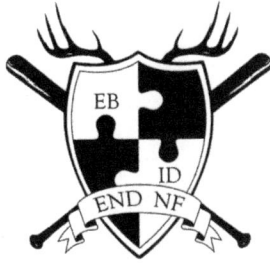

CHAPTER 1

The night before I was born, the smell of freshly popped popcorn filled the cool, crisp May air as my dad, Rick Brown, stepped up to the plate, confidently locked eyes with the pitcher, and with the tip of his bat pointed to the fences. The pitcher lobbed a softball to the plate, and the ping of ball to bat pierced the air. I guess it's thanks to him that I have a love of sports and the kind of tenacity one needs to win—both in the game and in life.

When I was a kid, I was terrified of many things, especially bees and the dark. Every night, I left my closet light on with the doors open. Sometimes, I'd even beg my mom to lie down with me. Her head would be at the foot of my bed, so I'd grab and hold her legs. Often when I would wake up and she wasn't there, I would run across the house to my parents' room to be with them.

My favorite song back then was a VeggieTales song called "God Is Bigger." He was bigger than the dark, which seemed so big and scary back then. I guess a lot of kids are scared of the dark, probably because they're scared of the unknown. I'm not scared of the dark anymore, maybe because I've had to deal with the unknown for a long time now—that's life with neurofibromatosis.

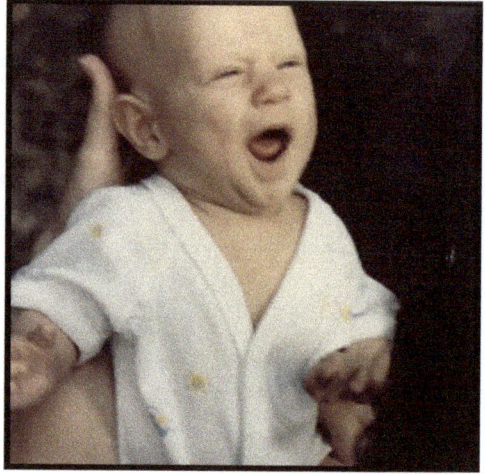

If you think that's hard to pronounce, try living with it! Actually, we just call it by its abbreviation, NF. NF has three types: NF1, NF2, and schwannomatosis. You can inherit NF from a parent (there's a 50 percent chance of passing it to your offspring if you have it), or you can get it from a spontaneous mutation like I did.

NF1 is the most common, occurring in 1 in 3,000 births worldwide regardless of race or gender. It can cause a loss of eyesight—some have to have their eyes removed because of tumors behind them—loss of limbs, and cancer.

NF2, which I have, is the next most common form of NF. It occurs in 1 in 25,000 births worldwide regardless of race or gender. It also can cause loss of eyesight, hearing, and limbs, and it can cause cancer and loss of balance.

The recently discovered form schwannomatosis is rare and affects 1 in 40,000 births worldwide. Not much is known about this form of NF.

Since I have NF2, I will focus on that type in this book.

Since 2008, I have had five major brain surgeries, lost my hearing, and developed facial weakness. I have limited vision, and my eyes do not produce moisture like they should. My left eye has an ulcer and is also sewn three-fourths of the way shut. My vocal cords are paralyzed, which makes it difficult for me to talk and for others to understand me.

For some reason, I drool, especially when I'm warm or hot. My mouth gets really dry, despite the drool. I can't swallow well, so all my liquids must be thickened to keep me from choking. The drooling is worse when I eat, so I wear a bib to avoid a messy shirt. I used to hate to go out to eat because I feared what others might think of me, but I got over that because this is who I am.

NF has taken a toll on my physical appearance. I used to go to the gym five days a week, but now I'm lucky to go twice a week. I prefer to use my left hand for almost everything because my right hand is uncoordinated. I can still move it, but I can't control it well. I use American Sign Language a lot to communicate, but it's very difficult, and I'm still learning. If you had asked my dad before 2013, he would have told you that my handwriting looked like chicken scratch. Now, I can't even manage that. It takes all I have to make a legible *EB*.

I have tumors in my left hand. We went to see a hand specialist, but he said he would not try to remove them because if the surgeon cut one of the many nerves in my hand, I could lose hand function.

I have a tumor on my spine and tumors on my feet and ankles, requiring me to wear foot drop braces to keep my feet straight. I don't have my balance, so I need a wheelchair to get around.

None of this stops me from trying to improve myself and to inspire those around me. It'll be very interesting to see how NF affects me in the years to come.

Isn't it comforting to know that God is bigger than anything we face (John 16:33)? Jesus tells us he has overcome the world. If we have accepted Jesus as Lord, the Holy Spirit lives inside us. We are told in 1 John 4:4, "You, dear children, are from God and have overcome them, because the one who is in you is greater than the one who is in the world."

Fear not, friends! Don't fear for me, and if you know Christ as your Savior, don't fear for yourself either.

My journey with NF started with a series of seemingly unconnected medical episodes that gave no hint of the challenges that lay ahead. I was in third grade when I had a fibroma, a benign tumor, removed from the back of my head. The doctor told us I could have it taken off if it bothered me. So that's what we did. Little did we know how much that one bump would mark a change in our lives. The surgery left me with a bald spot. My doctor told me to tell anyone who asked that I had my "memory expansion chip" removed. (I think I'll be needing that back!)

Later that year, I had my wisdom teeth removed, and I also had a growth on my tongue removed. The pathology report said that I needed to be evaluated for something called neurofibromatosis, but I wasn't. So, we went on with our lives like normal. Nobody in my family has NF, so we really didn't give it much thought.

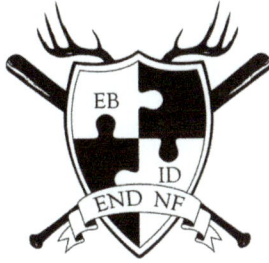

CHAPTER 2

Like my dad, I've always loved baseball.

My maternal grandma, Ma-Ma, loved the Atlanta Braves, so during the summers there were lots of Braves baseball games on TV. Chipper Jones was my favorite player. I even named a dog after him.

I've never seen a happier baseball player than Andruw Jones, Chipper's teammate. He always had a smile on his face. The camera zoomed in on him once after he struck out, and while walking back to the dugout, he was grinning ear to ear.

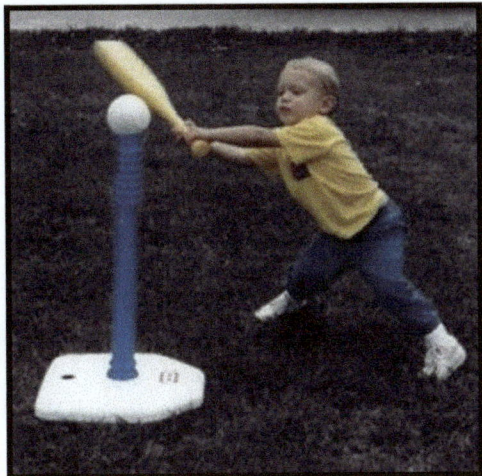

Growing up, I played recreation baseball every year. I played fall ball one year, but there was a problem. I couldn't catch a fly ball. The coaches stuck me in the outfield, which worked pretty well until the batters got big enough to hit the ball that far. I actually received the "Hustle" Award once. My guess is that it was like a participation trophy: "We know you aren't very good, but we see you trying!"

I also played football every year I could because I just loved to compete. My parents filmed the football games for the coaches in recreation league ball. Once, my dad and I were watching the films, and he wanted to show me how to properly engage and block someone. He got so into it that he picked me up and threw me onto a table. We broke the table, but he got his point across!

I thought I was decent in basketball, too, so I tried out when I was in seventh grade. We were warming up on the floor with some sit-ups. I was trying really hard: one, two, three, FART! The coach looked my way. "I hear you Ethan!" he yelled. Maybe I shouldn't have tried quite *that* hard.

But it seemed to all work out. At the end of try-outs, I was handed a letter saying I had made the team. I was ecstatic! On top of the world! I told everybody I had made the team!

The next day, the coach told me he had given me the wrong letter by mistake. I had not made the team. He told me I could be manager if I wanted to. I was crushed. I cried a good bit and was mad at the coach for a few days. But he was my homeroom teacher that year, so I couldn't stay mad at him, even if I had wanted to. I let it go pretty quickly and decided to run track to work on my speed. Tron Jackson, who had played running back at the University of Georgia, was my coach, and he knew a good bit about speed. (As an aside, Tron's daughter, Daysha, later married C. J. Spiller.) Unfortunately, the speed drills didn't work out for me; no matter how hard I tried, I was still slow. In the 40-yard dash, I ran a blazing 5.6!

By eighth grade, I was too old for recreation league sports, so it was either play for my school or sit at home. Because I loved football so much, I decided to play for my school. I was used to leaving school and downing a snack—which usually included a Little Debbie cake (or two), sometimes a sandwich, or both. One day, I ate a Smucker's peanut butter and jelly sandwich before practice and learned quickly that wasn't a good idea. I puked my guts out.

You could always spot me when we stretched. I had balance problems and was always stumbling or falling over. You could say that I played guard and tackle: I guarded the water bucket and tackled anyone who came near it.

On a serious note, in eighth grade, I won the Best Offensive Lineman Award. Either I was the best, or the coaches didn't have much to choose from. That's still up for debate!

I also tried out for basketball again and actually made the team. There was a new coach, so he didn't know what had happened the previous year. I also did shot-put for the track team that year. The guys told me I could run in the fat boy relay. That was enticing to me because I thought I could actually win that event.

When the high school football coaches were at the award ceremony for spring sports, I'm pretty sure I heard one coach say, "That's Ethan Brown," and the other say, "Gosh!" I was around five eleven and weighed about 170 pounds at the time, and I was still growing! I grew almost an inch, added weight, and slimmed down, but I was still slow. So, I stuck with the line for high school football.

I had a decent enough freshman season to earn varsity scrimmage time, and I was on the varsity kickoff return team. On a cool fall night, my school, Liberty High School, was playing Pickens High School, one of our biggest rivals. We won the coin toss and elected to kick off as our whole sideline chanted, "Hit squad!" several times.

After Pickens scored on a quick offensive drive, I went out on the field as "Kernkraft 400" by Zombie Nation was playing. I jumped up and down and bobbed my head to the music trying to psych myself up for what I hoped was to be a teeth-shattering block.

The kicker looked both ways to make sure his unit was ready, and after running five yards, put a booming kick to the ball. I started my run back to form a wall for the returner to run behind. He caught it, so I turned around to start blocking. When I turned, two opposing players were yards away from me and my angle on both of them was awful. I had no shot at hitting them, so I hoped that by throwing an arm out to catch one of them, maybe I'd slow him down. I completely missed, and when I got back to the sideline, I received an earful from an irate coach. He hit the top of my helmet and yelled, "What was that?!" I wasn't good at answering questions under pressure, so I said, "I don't know," which obviously wasn't the case. You can't justify yourself to adults. Needless to say, I didn't go back into the game and ultimately lost my job. We lost that game and only won one game that whole season.

One of our most memorable games that year was Liberty against Easley High School, another big rival. At that time, Geico Insurance was running an advertisement that said switching to them was so easy a caveman could do it. The students from Easley came to the game dressed as cavemen and hung up a huge sign that read, "Liberty is so easy to beat a caveman could do it." They took the sign down at halftime as the score was tied at 13 to 13. The game went into overtime. They scored and converted a two-point play. Then we got the ball and scored a few plays later. Our stadium was rocking, and our sideline was jumping and high-fiving. We ended up losing the game 21–20.

* * *

Usually, you hear of student athletes struggling to keep their grades up. I'm blessed to say that wasn't a problem for me. In the fall of 10th grade, I made the A/B honor roll and received Scholar Athlete status from my school. I was practicing football until six o'clock most days, playing a game on Thursday nights, then dressing for varsity games on Friday. I am proud to say that I was not only an athlete, but a scholar athlete. That said, I hated to read unless I was reading about sports. But my English class had to read *To Kill a Mockingbird*, and I can honestly say that it is one of my favorites to this day.

In the spring of 10th grade, I competed in a regional weight lifting meet at West-Oak High School. It was a junior varsity meet, so I felt pretty good about things. Squat was my best event as I was lifting 315 pounds compared to 180 pounds on bench press. Although I won my weight class, I finished third due to an error.

The top three athletes got to compete in the statewide meet. An athlete who later played football at Rutgers was in my weight class, along with players who played their college ball at the University of South Carolina. I finished 19th out of 21 that day. They counted the 40-yard dash, so a guy who squat 225 but ran faster finished ahead of me.

I also become very interested in lifting weights, and I tried to gain weight. I even had a sheet of paper from my strength coach taped to my bedroom door about how to gain weight.

My dad worked out a lot after high school and could squat 500 pounds. I was headed in that direction while I was still in school. My squat max jumped 100 pounds or more in one year of high school.

Looking back, I think that playing sports all my life has helped me cope with my NF. I'm a fighter: I fight to win, even when I know the odds are against me.

* * *

By the spring of my sophomore year, I started waking up with headaches so bad that it felt like my right eye would pop out of my head. I was told it was sinus pressure because nothing had shown up on the scans I'd previously had.

The pain would only go away after a hot shower, but my dad told me I had to stop the showers. The pain persisted, so by early summer, the doctors finally did a scan with contrast, and my world was turned upside down.

A longtime family friend was the radiology department manager at our local clinic. After checking in for my radiology appointment, I walked down a dimly lit hall to take my seat. When my mom saw her radiologist friend crying, she asked her if everything was okay.

"You know, this job can be tough sometimes," she replied. We soon learned that she was crying over the tumor she'd found in my brain. This woman has a son five days older than me.

I called my head coach to tell him the result. He didn't answer, so I left a voicemail asking for him to call me back. He called a few minutes later, not knowing anything was going on. I paused for a moment, thinking over everything. Then I said it: "Well, Coach, I have a brain tumor." As you can imagine, he was graveyard silent. He finally said, "I'll be praying for you."

I would need all the prayers I could get.

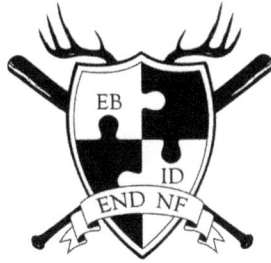

CHAPTER 3

The doctors told me that I had neurofibromatosis type 2 (NF2), a genetic disorder characterized by noncancerous tumors on the nerves that transmit balance and sound impulses from the inner ear to the brain. They told me I had to stop lifting weights. I was disappointed because I knew that if muscles aren't being exercised, you lose them.

After finding out I had NF, the Children's Tumor Foundation sent me a few things: two bracelets imprinted with "Solve the NF Puzzle," a tote bag, and a few more items. CTF would become a big part of my life, but I didn't know it then.

I tried to finish the 11th grade at my school, but with the effects of medication, numerous doctor visits, and my declining health (my right eye was shutting, the tumor was compressing my brain stem, and the medication was rough), everything seemed to overwhelm me. So, I went on homebound study.

I swelled up to 204 pounds while I was taking medical steroids.

The doctor told us, "You would be dead if we hadn't found this when we did." I was kind of at a loss for words. I thought back to all the episodes I had before, like the benign tumor when I was a kid and the tumor on my tongue. Once, I had a tumor in my breast, but the doctor had said it was breast tissue that should go away (I still have that tumor). I had been told that all these issues were nothing to be concerned with.

That football season began without me. There is nothing more painful than watching your teammates lay it all on the line and knowing you should be out there on the field with them. Coach gave me a football that everyone signed. What stood out is something that he often told me: "Fight the good fight." It's actually a verse in the Bible, 1 Timothy 6:12. I'm still trying to fight the good fight. Every day is a fight, especially those days when I don't even want to get out of bed.

The team ended up winning four games that season. The school let my parents and me watch the games from our car, and they even raised money for me by selling wristbands in red and black, our school colors, with my name and football jersey number, 65, on them. I received so much stuff from them that we had to put everything on a huge dining table in the kitchen. What I thought was most helpful was a bowl full of quarters for the vending machines at the hospital.

My parents and I saw two doctors, one in Greenville, South Carolina, and one out of state. The out-of-state doctor's assistant told us I'd have to wait until December or later to have surgery, but that he really felt that the surgeon who operated first would have the best chance of getting the tumor. The surgeon in Greenville said that we couldn't wait—that the surgery needed to be done as soon as possible. In his view, it would be much better to have the surgery done locally, and since I was in a lot of pain, my parents asked me whether I could wait. I told them I couldn't, and they scheduled the surgery, much to the delight of the doctor here.

Before my surgery, the doctor said they needed to do an awake procedure through my groin. It was a procedure to apply aneurysm clips to see if I could function with less blood flow. The woman talking to me during the procedure told Mom she had to sit down because she got sick from the size of the needles they were using.

The morning of my surgery, my school let students who wanted to see me be late for school. My parents rolled me into the waiting room, and I saw about a dozen or more smiling classmates. The visits from schoolmates didn't stop after that morning, and that meant a lot to me. I was told that so many people came that they had to move my family and friends to another waiting room.

The surgery lasted nine hours, and I came out of it fine. The doctors said they got what they needed.

The doctor performing the surgery had told us that they were going to make only a small incision and that we didn't need to cut my hair. When I woke from surgery, my head was half-shaved and had a huge incision the shape of a crescent moon, held together with staples. My mom was so horrified that she turned and ran. The nurses had to stop her!

My football coach went to church with a few players from Clemson, so after about a week, he thought it was time to get a few Tigers to come see me. It totally surprised me! I was told I had some visitors coming, and it made my night to see two

Clemson guys, Willy Korn and Xavier Dye, with my football coach. They brought me a few items, but the thing that stood out to me was a note that read:

To: Ethan Brown,

I want you to know I will have you in my prayers and I want you to keep your faith positive because our Lord and Savior will have His hands on you, and everything will be fine. I hope to come see you soon.

Your #1 Fan,
C. J. Spiller

Spiller had been hurt in practice earlier, so he was unable to come with the others. He was an NCAA running back who later went on to play professional football. At Clemson, he shared the backfield with James Davis, and that duo earned the name Thunder & Lightning. Spiller ran a 4.3 in the 40-yard dash, making him the Lightning. They had a saying: "If the Thunder doesn't get you, the Lightning will!"

When my mom got a call from a restricted number, she handed me the phone, saying it was for me. I answered, and a voice asked if this was Ethan Brown.

"Yes, it is. Who is this?"

The voice said, "This is Tommy Bowden."

I smiled from ear to ear, and we talked for a few minutes. Bowden was head football coach at Clemson University. His father is the legendary Florida State coach Bobby Bowden.

I was also visited by two Clemson basketball players.

One of my dad's friends told Dad that I would be getting something from coaches of teams that I didn't even root for, and he was right. I received a signed picture from South Carolina's Steve "the Head Ball Coach" Spurrier. It said the Gamecocks were pulling for me. My dad snickered, "They might be pulling for you, but you're not pulling for them."

I also received an envelope from the University of Georgia; I thought it was just a signed picture, but I got more than I bargained for:

Dear Ethan,

I recently heard of your illness and hope this letter finds you on the road to recovery.

*I tell our Bulldog football players to work as
hard as they can every day and not to give
up in a game no matter how tired they are.
We call this "finishing the drill." I know you
will do the same as you fight to beat this
disease.*

*The Bulldogs and I are pulling for you. God
bless.*

Sincerely,
Mark Richt

In a few days I was able to go home, but I wasn't
any better. My eye was still shut and didn't move. I
was in constant pain despite all the pain medication,
so my dad looked for other options. That led us to
Duke University.

Before we headed to Duke for my next major
brain surgery, the doctor at home in Greenville,
South Carolina, told me I needed to start learning
sign language because I was going to be deaf after
the surgery. The doctors at Duke had to go through
my ear to get the tumor, and the doctors in Greenville didn't want to do a cochlear implant until after
the surgery. But when we got to Duke, the doctor
said he would do the implant then so that after the

surgery in December, I wouldn't be deaf.

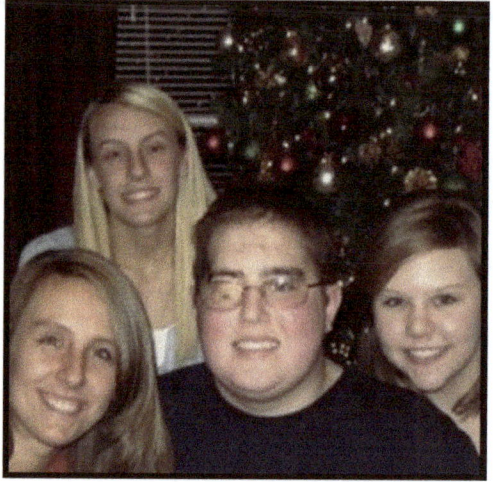

So, in November 2008, I had the cochlear implant surgery. After having the implant put in, it took a while for my brain to get used to it. Initially, I was hearing two voices—my natural hearing and the hearing from the device. The implant picked up sound slower than my natural hearing. It felt like I was listening to Alvin and the Chipmunks.

I cried, devastated that I'd never hear things as they should sound. My parents tried to comfort me by saying that my nurse had a friend with an implant, and she could talk on the phone. It was hard to be comforted by that. I was 16 and scared, facing the dark unknown. As time went by, I rarely used the implant unless I was forced to.

The brain surgery at Duke was scheduled for December 11, 2008. As it drew closer, a church friend helped us fund the trip with a hot dog benefit. The woman who put it together told my mom they were planning to sell 10,000 plates! My mom told her that she was crazy, but she replied, "I'm telling you; we're going to sell 10,000 plates."

My family got Dan Scott, former host of Cruise Control on WCCP-FM 104.9, to mention the benefit on his show. The benefit was to feature a silent auction. The words *silent auction* didn't click with me at first. My football coach brought a helmet to be auctioned off, so I decided to look at the sheet to see what people were bidding on it. Upon seeing the sheet, I yelled out, "Uh-oh! My old youth pastor was outbid!"

Everyone stopped and looked at me. The higher bidder looked at me with a finger over her mouth. She was my former PE teacher, so I hushed because she was the type of person who meant business. It was pretty embarrassing once I figured out what "silent auction" meant. I still laugh at myself and shake my head.

A lot of items were donated for the silent auction. I had my eye on one of them, though. Someone had donated a signed baseball and cards by Taylor Harbin, who had played second base at Clemson before being selected by the Arizona Diamondbacks in the 2007 Major League Baseball draft. Later, he was hired as an assistant coach at Furman University.

Someone gave my cousin Kristen a hundred dollars and told her to bid on whatever I wanted. She went all in on my favorite, and I came away from the benefit with the Taylor Harbin items.

Many people attended the benefit to show their support: people from school, church, the community, and even people I didn't know. A small local college basketball team came and presented me with a check and a jersey.

"I'm from Seneca," one elderly man told me. (Seneca is about 45 minutes away.) "You don't know me, but I felt led to come here and give you this money."

We ended up raising $12,000, and the cooks had to keep going back to the store for more supplies. A few days later, we headed to Duke.

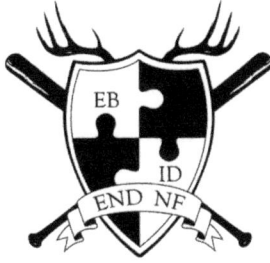

CHAPTER 4

On December 10, 2008, my parents and I set off for Duke University Hospital and the Millennium Hotel in Durham, North Carolina. The Greenville Hospital System oncology clinic near my home has a foundation called the Ellis Mayfield Foundation that pays for patients and their families to stay at the Millennium. The family who started the foundation had a son with an aggressive brain tumor, and they stayed at that hotel while he was undergoing treatment. Having a place to stay while we were at Duke was a blessing because, although the benefit raised quite a bit of money, we didn't know how long I would have to stay in Durham. Another blessing was that the clinic gave us food and gas cards for our trip up.

I was told the surgery would take 24 hours total, scheduled over two days in two 12-hour shifts, starting December 11. During surgery, the surgical team would go through my ear canal and get as much of the tumor as possible. Although this would destroy my hearing nerve, causing me to be deaf, it was the safest and best approach to get the tumor.

It scared me to high heaven to think I might be asleep 24 hours. I asked my parents what would happen if I pooped while I was sleeping. My mom reassured me that she was sure the staff had experience in this area and would take care of it. The thought still unnerved me. How embarrassing would that be!

But comforts abounded. My mom, who is a business manager, had received a painting from her boss to take with us to Duke. It is called *Chief of the Medical Staff* and shows Jesus guiding a surgeon's hand in an operating room. Mom had told her boss that I really liked the painting, so he took it off his wall and gave it to her. I made it the background on my phone, so I looked at it often.

The morning of my surgery, before heading back to the operating room, I quickly showed the picture to a doctor on the team. My dad told him, "There's going to be an extra person in the room."

The surgery lasted only nine hours. The doctors said they had gotten what they needed and that my body could not handle any more surgery.

I woke up from my surgery in a pitch-black room, scared and convinced I was dead.

I don't know whether the nurse's name was Beth, or whether I just chose that name. But I started yelling, "Beth! Beth!" The next morning, I woke to see what looked like a different woman in the room with me, and I asked, "Who are you?"

She replied that she was Beth.

Angry, I said, "No, you're not!"

To this day, I have no idea who the first woman was—probably a nurse who heard me calling out and came to calm me down.

Turns out, all the medication in my system was making me confused and angry. I was in ICU, and I didn't know that I was still catheterized when I told my parents I had to pee. When they didn't respond, I yelled, "I said I got to pee!"

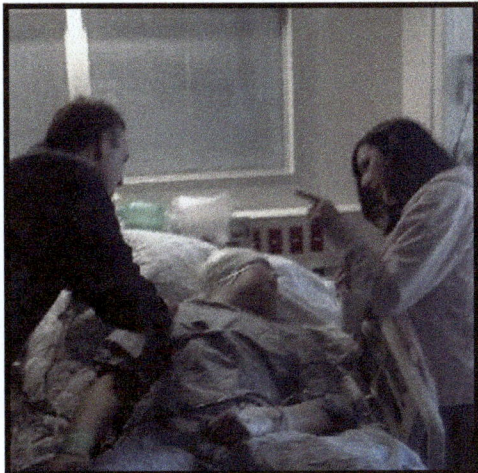

My mom hushed me, told me a baby was next door, and said not to be so mean.

When it was time for Mom and Dad to go back to the hotel, I whined that I didn't want to be left alone in the hospital. They argued that there wasn't a bed for Mom to sleep on, but I kept on whining, so she stayed.

She started out sitting in a chair but eventually crawled into bed with me.

My incision was itching, so I lifted my hand to lightly rub it, but Mom caught my arm as I was moving it toward my scalp. I told her that it was itching badly and that I needed to scratch it, but she caught my hand again. After she rolled over, I slowly moved my hand toward my head again, but she turned over to face me, so I stopped where I was. After watching her a few minutes, I decided she was asleep, so I very slowly started the upward motion again. Just when I thought the coast was clear, she opened her eyes. I rushed my hand up to my head. She grabbed my hand and started wrestling with me to stop my scratching. After a few minutes, she called a nurse, and the two of them overpowered me.

In a day or two I was transferred to a regular room. I kept asking my parents whether I would be home for Christmas. All I wanted was to be home with them; I didn't need anything else. My family came to visit me often, and that meant a lot because it was almost a five-hour drive. The stay at Duke wasn't bad at all, but the distance and not having as many visitors as I did after my previous surgery made me eager to go home.

What was lacking in quantity was made up in quality. Members of the Carolina Hurricanes, who are frequent visitors to the Duke Children's Hospital, came by, signed a poster, and gave me a small stuffed team animal. The mascot from the Durham Bulls made a visit as well, signing his Wool E. Bull baseball card. The hospital therapy dogs also paid me a visit. I'm a sucker for dogs, so when the staff asked whether I wanted them to come in to see me, I said yes without hesitation.

During my surgery, the doctors took fat from my stomach to put inside my ear before sewing it shut. Normally, if you stick a finger in an ear, it'll move a bit. My right ear is not like that. If you try to place your finger in my ear, it just stops.

I knew they were going to do it, but I somehow forgot I had a tube hanging from my stomach to catch blood and fluid that drained from the area.

I told my mom I had to use the bathroom, and I jerked the covers off me not thinking. Whatever fluids were inside the tube spilled out onto the white bed sheets. I thought my mom would pass out.

I also had a tube in my back draining fluid off my spine from a spinal tap. I started to the bathroom with Mom, but I lost it there in the middle of my room. I was so embarrassed. I almost cried, and I apologized again and again.

My nurse came and told me they were going to remove the drain from my lower back and that I could have it removed with a shot to numb the area or have it done without the shot. I chose doing it without the shot, and that was a huge mistake. The pain was so bad that I screamed.

I had a scratch on my right eye, so an eye doctor put a plastic bubble on it to keep moisture in and prevent me from rubbing my eye. Most of the doctors and nurses I had at Duke were University of North Carolina fans, and they decorated the tape holding the bubble in place with flowers and University of North Carolina drawings. There was a video game console in the room, and I asked if they had a baseball game.

When a patient in a room next to mine was discharged, he left a pill-shaped balloon that had *Get*

Well written on it and told the nurse to give it to someone who needed it. The balloon looked a little like a bat, and since she knew I loved baseball, my nurse gave it to me. Then she tossed me a roll of tape, telling me to pitch it to her. I asked if I heard her right because I'd always been told you don't throw a ball or play baseball inside (unless you're the Toronto Blue Jays, but they're from Canada, so I guess, they get a pass). She told me I heard right, so I tossed the tape to the batter. She hit a homer with the balloon "bat" and circled the room as if she were rounding the bases. I asked her if we could take a selfie or get a picture together. She said, "Sure!" and jumped into bed with me! Another worker came into the room while she was there beside me. She looked at the nurse like, "What are you doing?" The nurse quickly got up and said, "We were just taking a picture."

Another nurse came in, and as she leaned over my bed, I noticed her Tweety Bird earrings and told her I liked them. Later, she brought me a Tweety Bird ornament for my Christmas tree. It had a button that made Tweety say, "Merry Christmas!"

The oncology clinic back home has a foundation that gives its patients one item they ask for. I asked for a laptop so that while I was at Duke, I could go on YouTube and listen to the song "You Never Let Go" by Matt Redman (I was not completely deaf at this point). I was definitely in the midst of a storm, and that song, along with the painting of Jesus in the operating room, comforted me.

The doctors usually came to my room early in the morning at the start of their day. One morning, my surgeon and his assistant came in and started talking to my dad. When I told them that I could hear the conversation, the doctor said my nerve must not be fully dead yet. I still had my cochlear implant but couldn't wear it at night; this was early morning before I put it on.

He then told my dad I was doing well and would get to go home soon.

With a huge smile and triumph in my voice, I looked at the assistant and shouted, "Ha! No more waking up to you!"

Dad jumped in and said, "I wouldn't be too happy. She's pretty."

I was just kidding, but I also just really wanted to go home!

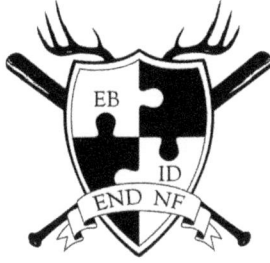

CHAPTER 5

When I got home, I complained to my mom that my nose was hurting. After looking inside my nose, she gasped and said she thought I had cancer. Besides making me gain weight, the steroids I was on had also eaten a hole in my nose. I now have a deviated septum. On the bright side, I was losing the weight I had gained, and my right eye started to open.

I spent some time at my grandparents' house before Christmas. One day, I was listening to Dan Scott's sports talk radio show. He was raising money for a family for the holidays. He repeatedly mentioned that people should come see them at the store where they were broadcasting. Pa-pa asked me if I wanted to go. Since I had nothing better to do, I agreed, and my cousin Kristen, my grandpa, and I set off to the location.

"You might get on the radio," Pa-pa said.

Something to know about Pa-pa: He's not the most careful at times. Every winter, he would take me trout fishing in the mountains. The road up was curvy, and he'd use both lanes. I can still hear Ma-Ma yelling, "Gary!" My parents used to tell me to look out for him and be sure he didn't get hurt. Funny how things work out. Now he's looking out for me.

When we got there, I slowly walked into the store with help on both sides to make sure I didn't fall. After we gave money to help, they put me on the air for a few minutes.

Dan said, "This is Ethan Brown joining us on the show; this is a young man we've talked a lot about as he was facing surgery at Duke. He came by with several members of his family to see us and basically walked in by himself. You're wearing a patch on your right eye. Are you going to get the sight back?"

"I have full sight in my eye. I just have a scratch on it," I said. "Duke patched it for a couple of days."

"How was the hospital food?"

"It was nasty!"

Dan laughed. "As it usually is! What's the one thing you missed doing?"

I said that I really missed school.

"Really? Never thought you'd say that, did you?"

"No. Just seeing everyone and having something to do. Yesterday my uncle brought a stack of cards from my high school this thick."

"He's holding his fingers three to four inches apart," Dan explained for the listening audience. "They say you don't know what you have until it's gone."

"That's right."

"What have the doctors told you? Have they said if you can play football again?"

"They haven't said anything yet, but if they clear me, I'm ready to go!"

Then he gave me a big surprise: "I'm going to make you a promise on the air, and Lee is recording us. We tried to make it happen this year but had some technical difficulties. If you're on the football field next year, we will do one of Liberty's games as our Friday Night High School Game of the Week, but you have to be on the field. I don't know how it'll happen, but we will make it happen. Is it a deal?"

"It's a deal," I said. "It's going to happen."

I had gone to the store to give money for the family who Dan was raising money for, but then people came to the store to see, greet, or give me money. "You don't know me, but I was listening to the show and felt led to come and give you this money," someone told me.

That was just the beginning of my brush with fame. Before Christmas, I was interviewed by Bob Castello, a former front-page reporter for the sports section in the largest newspaper in the Upstate. He told my whole story, and I was able to share the truth of Jeremiah 29:11: "'For I know the plans I have for you,' declares the LORD, 'plans to give you hope and a future.'" God has plans for me, including my NF.

Later, I was also interviewed by News 7 for a television broadcast in the Greenville, South Carolina, area. They gave my story again, and since it was around Christmas, the interviewer said that the greatest gift of the season was on the couch—meaning me!

***

After Christmas, I continued with my homebound schooling using a microphone to help me communicate. The microphone I used had a 70/30 split—I heard 70 percent of the teacher and 30 percent of the background noise. It was a pretty cool device. It came with an audio cable so that I could listen to music without having to be in the same room as my iPod. My homebound teacher was excellent. She often reviewed my work and nudged me to double-check my work when she caught errors.

I was determined to play football again. Every day, I did the therapy exercises Duke had given me, and I was making good progress. My parents also took me to outpatient therapy. My balance and strength improved greatly. I was walking by myself by late January 2009.

My football coach delivered a letter to me that said that I had been invited to the High School Sports Report (HSSR) Fall Awards Banquet. I had been nominated for the Tommy Mangum Valor Award—the state Courage Award that is presented to an athlete who participated in a fall sport despite major physical injury or trauma. I won the award.

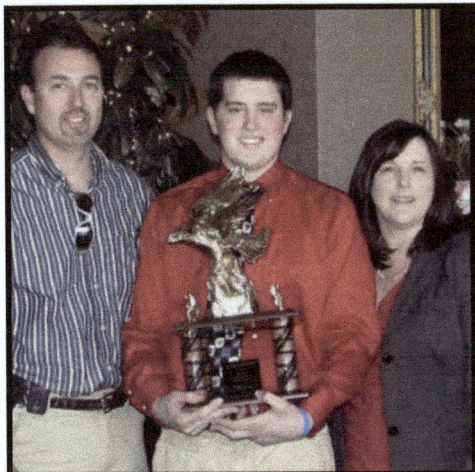

The key speaker was a football coach for a big school. During his speech, he said that we have 90,000 thoughts a day, and

90 percent of those thoughts are what we thought yesterday. He said that when he recruits new players, he doesn't have to hear them talk because their actions speak for them.

Now that I'm deaf, I can tell you how true that really is. I pick up on everything that people's body language gives off. Before I became completely deaf, someone from the school district commented that she had observed that deaf people notice things that other students don't.

After the HSSR awards banquet, my parents and I had to go to Duke for a postoperative visit. We sat in the room waiting for my surgeon while I watched football videos, eagerly waiting the okay to play on the field again.

The doctors came into the room to meet us—minus one who was in Japan. We made small talk before discussing the surgery. Then I asked the doctors whether I could play football again. They said that if I felt like I could play and if my body could handle the strain, then yes.

Then the doctors turned to my parents and said, "Doctor F [the doctor in Japan] was furious when he got inside your son's head. The previous surgeon in

Greenville butchered your son. Fortunately, everything looks okay, but that stroke on the brain—"

The doctor didn't get any further because Mom jumped in. "Stroke! What stroke? We didn't know about that."

The doctors said the clips the Greenville surgeon had inserted weren't necessary; I'm now stuck with them. Apparently, the surgery to insert the clips damaged parts of my brain. It was frustrating to learn, but the doctors were reassuring.

"Will it affect him?" Mom asked.

Their reply was reassuring. "No, it's on a part of the brain that won't be affected."

After we left Duke, I received more practice with my implant microphone, and I was ready for the next school year. I finished that year with all As, and before I knew it, I was preparing to play football my senior year.

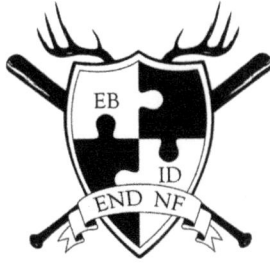

CHAPTER 6

It was early fall, and that summer had gone well. I weighed 180 pounds and was squatting about 275 pounds. A lot of people did not expect me to make it that far or even play football again, but there I was ready to play.

Before the season started, Bob Castello, the *Greenville News* sports reporter, came to a practice to interview Coach Curtis Middleton and me. He asked how it felt for me to be working out again and in the weight room.

"Before I got sick, I was in a weight lifting competition, so I was thinking I was strong. But getting back in the weight room, I realized I was weak, and it was bad. People were squatting three hundred fifty pounds, and I was doing one hundred," I said.

As I recall it, Coach Middleton summed up my progress in words to this effect: "Just the work ethic he's had in the weight room is incredible. I mean he went from doing two hundred fifty to two hundred seventy-five pounds down to just the bar, and he didn't really care. He was just glad to be in there and working. He would turn around and encourage the other boys and get on them about going lower in their squats and helping with their form. He had so much self-confidence and self-awareness of where he was at."

Then Castello asked about my role on the team.

"I'm working myself hard, but I believe that if I could just get in the weight room more and work more, I will get better. Right now, I'm starting field goal snapping. I mean, I accept that role, but I really want to start doing a whole lot more for the team," I said.

Before the season started, someone from Laurens High School, where Coach Middleton had previously coached, asked me if I would be interested in speaking to their Fellowship of Christian Athletes. I was excited because I had no idea what I was supposed to do with my life and the thought of possibly being a speaker was exciting.

I was supposed to be dead, but I wasn't. God had been so good to me, and now I could tell my story. I was nervous because this was my first time speaking to people I didn't know well. It didn't go too well. I had a runny nose and sniffled a lot. Having a microphone near my mouth carried the sniffle sound throughout the gym. I got my words mixed up. I meant to say, "You Never Let Go" by Matt Redman, but it came out, "You Never Lose Faith." Coach Middleton even asked me to lift my arms to let him see my sweat stains. He could tell I was nervous, and he talked a few minutes for me.

The first game of the season came quickly. I had a lot to prove that night, I thought as I applied my eye black stickers, on which I had written "Psalm 23:4." A lot of people didn't think I would play football again, and I wanted to prove myself on the field.

Radio announcer Dan Scott made good on his promise, and he and his broadcast team were there to broadcast the game.

We'd played this team the year before. It was a back-and-forth game that we lost by a few points. Before the game, a radio show host asked me to call in and give my score prediction, and I told them I thought we'd win in a close game.

The stage was set: Liberty High School versus Christ Church Episcopal School, Friday Night High School Game of the Week!

As we were warming up, the coach from Christ Church ran over and handed my position coach a note that read:

To Ethan Brown: My son is #11. Please don't hurt him.

It felt great to feel strong and know that other people thought I was strong! The stands were packed with fans, including some of my family. I was a team captain for that game, and all the blood from practices, sweat in the weight room, and the tears of wishing I were playing were about to pay off. I was pumped to be out on the field again.

Before I knew it, we were down 7–0, and it only got worse from there. I was the starting field goal snapper, but we did not score until almost the last quarter.

The coaches put me on defense. My family has a picture of me being engaged with a blocker and throwing the guy down. The only problem was that the ball carrier ran right beside us, and I missed an easy tackle. I made up for it later.

After the game, a rush of people found me on the field, including the sideline reporter. Forgetting that I was deaf, he asked, "How'd it feel to hear the crowd when you got in?" Smiling from ear to ear, I hesitated for a second before saying, "Oh, it was awesome!" We talked for a few minutes before I had to get on the bus to go back to my school. I was stoked. Even though we lost the game by 30 points or more, it was a personal win for me.

A few weeks went by, and I was not playing much, if at all. We were losing a lot, and I stayed on the sideline. One day at school, I entered the coach's lounge and asked Coach Middleton if I could talk to him privately. He said, "Let's talk here."

With tears filling my eyes, I said, "I want to play. I've worked way too hard to just stand on the sideline."

"What do you want me to do?" he asked without hesitation. "Play the best eleven or what?" It was as if he had expected me to come to him. Turning to another coach, he said, "He's starting field goals, isn't he?"

I lowered my head and admitted that I wanted the best 11 to play. What I really wanted to say was, "Coach, we are terrible and get blown out every game—we hardly ever score. What difference would it make if I got to play now and then?" That had not gone the way I wanted it to, so I exited the room to get ready for practice.

A few weeks later, we were playing Carolina High School, and we were still winless. The coaches kept stressing that we just needed one win to make the playoffs. I wanted that win badly. Our mascot is a devil and the coach told us it's not the size of the devil in the fight but the size of the fight in the devil.

It was a back-and-forth game. We'd score; then they'd score. They had a stud defensive lineman who later played at Auburn, Devaroe "Jamal" Lawrence. He also played for NFL teams, and one of his coaches, Sam Kelly, who became a good friend of mine, took Jamal into his family.

Needless to say, we had a tough task that game. The game went into three overtime periods. I got to play in that game, but thanks to me and my bad point after touchdown snaps, we lost the game.

The following Monday, my coach asked if I wanted to go to the Greenville Touchdown Club to accept an award. Of course, I agreed to go. The quarterback and head coach of the team we played that last Friday also were there. Come to find out, I was the only player from outside that county to get an award. It was "For Overcoming Insurmountable Odds. To Play the Game He Loves the Most Which Is High School Football."

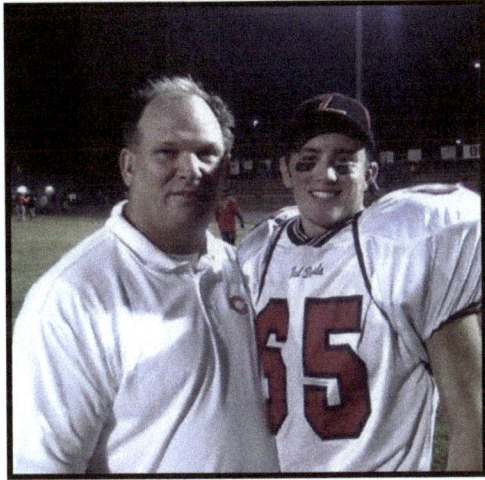

I had to give a short speech, so I summed up my story of tumors, surgeries, and determination:

> Three surgeries later, it is by God's grace that I stand before you and give Him all the praise and glory. He has granted me my prayer of being able to play football again. In many ways, football is like life, you never give up until the game is over. My body is weak, but my determination is strong.
>
> Everyone has fears. You face fear every single day of your life. When my doctor told me, "Son, you have a brain tumor,

and this is serious," I could have answered, "You know, I'm not ready for this. I'm scared!" But I was able to look him in the eye and say, "I'm not worried about this because I have God on my side."

Psalm 23:4 says, "Even though I walk through the darkest valley, I will fear no evil, for you are with me; your rod and your staff, they comfort me." Romans 8:31 says, "What, then, shall we say in response to these things? If God is for us, who can be against us?"

I'm telling you there is nothing in this life that you should fear. Nothing. If I could take on a brain tumor and look at the doctor and say, "I'm not afraid of this," there's nothing in your daily life that could be as bad as that.

Then I thanked my coaches and ended with my life verse, Jeremiah 29:11.

We finished that season winless, but I was asked to speak again, this time to a church youth group. A woman there was a teacher at my high school and had noticed the wristband I was wearing—the one my school had made to show support for me when I had the surgery in Greenville. The woman who had bid on the football helmet was also there with her husband.

I was thanking the school for all their help when her husband interrupted. "My son has a football helmet in his room," he said, "and wants to be just like you." I was thrilled to be an inspiration to others and a testimony of God's faithfulness.

I often got Facebook messages from a kid who ended his messages with, "The little #65," which was my football jersey number. I didn't realize it then, but now I understand that I was something of a hero to the town.

Romans 12:3 tells us not to think of ourselves "more highly than you ought." Just as we have one body with many members and each with different functions, so the members of the church in Christ make one body but with different gifts. I did not know what I was going to do with my life, but I knew I had a knack for speaking. In 10th grade I had a monotone teacher. Everything he said had the same even tone—even when he got excited about Guitar Hero having his favorite AC/DC songs and tried to jump around like a guitarist. It all sounded the same!

Can you imagine if we all had the same gifts? What a boring life to live.

One day, I went to my football locker and saw that it had already been unlocked. I looked in and found an envelope from Gallaudet University. They were recruiting me to play with the Bisons! It was only because I was deaf, but at the time, who cared? I sure didn't! After I told a few people that I'd received the letter, an assistant coach walked into the locker room and a teammate asked him, "Why didn't y'all tell him he was an All-American?"

The coach took the letter, looked it over, and with a confident voice said, "Yep, it's official."

I was on cloud nine. I had no clue how they knew about me. I had never contacted them, and I didn't even have a highlight video put together.

I did some research on the school, and it seemed like a decent fit for me because they not only offered the major that I wanted, but they also did video classes.

But my dad told me I had to go to Tri-County Tech in Pendleton, South Carolina, which was close to home. So, I only flirted with the idea of going to school in Washington, DC.

I messaged Willy Korn, whom I'd met a year prior. I wasn't sure whether he remembered who I was, but he invited me to a Clemson football game, where I was treated like a recruit and given a tour of the facilities, a group meeting with Coach Dabo, and more. It was a great experience, and at the end of the game, Dad and I went into the locker room with Willy to reveal who I was and ask whether he remembered me. I showed him a picture of us from when I was in the hospital. He was blown away and made us follow him to meet Xavier Dye.

Our high school season ended with zero wins. I won the Courage Award at our high school football awards ceremony. I finished 26th in my graduating class with a 3.875 GPA and was inducted into the Liberty High School Hall of Fame.

After my graduation, my grandmother's health started to decline rapidly. She was one of my biggest fans, and I learned how to fight from her by watching her battle arthritis and a lung disease that smokers get—even though she never smoked.

She and my parents taught me what being a true Christian is all about. She sat in the same spot every day with her Bible, making notes in the margins and underlining certain words or verses that stuck out to her. She had a lot of Christian books and a few commentaries by well-known and respected authors. If she wasn't reading her Bible or "resting her eyes," as she often said, you could hear her softly singing. Before the lung disease made breathing too difficult, she loved to sing and was a member of the church choir. Her favorite hymn was "Blessed Assurance."

Ma-Ma was on lots of medications—two of which were blood thinners and medical steroids. She bruised easily, and because she pushed the footrest of her recliner down with her legs, she eventually had bruises that turned into wounds.

As the home health-care nurses changed Ma-Ma's bandages, she would pray, "Jesus, please help me!"

One day in December, her wounds ruptured, and blood went everywhere in her bedroom. The ambulance came and rushed her to the hospital. Our family spent many nights in the hospital waiting room. People would bring us food as we waited for our time to go back to see her.

On December 24, I finally got to see her. It was almost midnight, and I stroked her hair, watching her struggle to breathe. "Please, I just want one more Christmas with you!" I was in her room as the clock struck 12:00 a.m., Christmas Day.

The next day, Dad and I were getting ready to take lunch to the hospital, so I hurried to feed my dog and play with him a bit. When I got in the car, Dad told me that Ma-Ma had died.

When we got to the hospital, Ma-Ma's sister was in the room with her. I stroked Ma-Ma's hair and kissed her head. "I just wanted to see you get better!" I cried.

Her sister put a hand on my shoulder and said, "But she saw you get better."

After her passing I wrote a poem:

What Does Ma-Ma Mean to Me?

Ma-Ma means strength.
Ma-Ma means courage.
Ma-Ma means faith that couldn't be shaken.
Ma-Ma means love.
Ma-Ma means my hero.
Ma-Ma means M&M's on Christmas.
This is what Ma-Ma means to me.

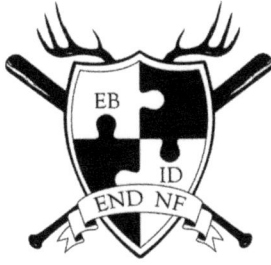

CHAPTER 7

Everything was quiet until 2012. I was actually doing pretty well for a while. The cochlear implant was working well, but as time went on, my hearing decreased. My church bought wireless headphones for me to use during services.

I was having MRIs every six months because the tumors were still growing. My parents asked the doctors at Duke about radiation, but they said they would rather start me on chemotherapy. If they performed surgery, they would have to remove my cochlear implant because it had been inserted through a tumor in my ear. Their goal was to try to preserve my hearing as long as possible; therefore, chemotherapy was our best option.

The only problem was that the chemo they wanted to use (Avastin) was still in trial and, therefore, not covered by my dad's awesome insurance. Avastin cost over $10,000 a treatment, so we did a lot of praying and waiting.

In February 2012, my treatment was approved for insurance. It was a huge relief because we obviously couldn't afford it otherwise. I was in my fifth semester at Tri-County Technical College where I was taking transfer classes in hopes of transferring to Clemson to pursue a degree in graphic communication. I had taken a college skills class and continued communicating with the professor on social media. He was a Clemson grad and was an academic advisor, so he offered to go to Clemson with me, show me around, and talk to professors we saw. He often told my class, "It's not the grades you make but the hands you shake."

We were able to talk to the department head, who sat down with me and explained which classes would be the easiest of the options I had to choose from. He said that it spoke highly of me for my former college skills teacher to come with me. Good grades and a good resume will only get you so far. It's the people you know who make the difference.

Sam Kelly emailed me that the Outdoor Dream Foundation (ODF) wanted to do something nice for me, but they had to hurry to get the papers filled out before I turned 21. ODF takes kids 21 or younger who have life-threatening or terminal illnesses on dream hunting or fishing trips. They also do local or other small trips for the kids.

One of the founders of this organization was the legendary T. L. Hanna football coach Herald Jones. If you have seen the movie *Radio*, his name should ring a bell. He and his family took in James Robert Kennedy—who was called Radio. His son Brad runs the ODF now, and I speak for all the families who have been on these trips: we are very thankful for the ODF.

I had never been hunting and didn't really know much about it, but each Sunday morning before church, I found and watched hunting shows. Those shows really bothered my mom because of how much the hunters whispered. I also didn't own any camouflage because Mom said it was redneck.

Sam told me to write on the paperwork that I wanted to hunt and then select three options. I didn't really know what I wanted to hunt, so I asked a hunting friend, who said to write down elk. I also selected mule deer and Columbian black-tail deer. A few weeks went by before the ODF approved my elk hunt and said they'd buy me a gun and outfit me with everything I needed.

In late May, my cousin Hailey asked if I'd be interested in speaking to a baseball team at Byrnes High School where her husband was in his first year as head coach.

I had a few speeches under my belt and had just taken a public speaking class, so I was more relaxed than I had been in previous years. Coach Maus introduced me and told the boys I drove over an hour to come speak to them.

I started out by asking them why they played baseball. "Is it throwing out that base runner trying to score in the bottom of the last inning? Is it getting a walk-off hit to win the game?" I then told them my story and emphasized how quickly a life can change. I was a seemingly healthy kid and then suddenly, I wasn't.

I showed them a video from when I had given a talk to my church congregation. It included pictures of me before, during, and after my surgeries. I ended with this: "If Coach Maus tells you to win a state championship, go win a state championship!"

They gave me a ball that everyone had signed. Hailey texted me afterward to say thank you and that my speech got her pumped, especially about winning a title. The team won the first game 2–0 but lost the last two games 6–5 and 4–3.

I was on Twitter Monday, June 4, and saw that the page Unashamed Athletes was retweeting prayer requests. Being a firm believer in prayer, I tweeted that I would be having chemo the next day and needed prayer because if the chemo I was taking didn't work, I would need brain surgery and would lose my hearing.

I wasn't expecting anyone to reply, but when I opened my Twitter app later, I had a notification from Ian Desmond, who played for the Washington Nationals.

> @ethanbrown65 just saw your prayer request through @athletes116 I will be praying for you. Stay strong my man, with God all is possible.

I followed him, and he followed back, so I sent him a direct message. I've always been taught to show respect to others, but after I called him "sir" for about the tenth time, he said, "You can call me Desi or Ian. Not sir—that's weird!"

As soon as I read that, I thought to myself, *"Yes, sir!"*

He went on to say that I'd made impressive progress. "Do you get a sense of accomplishment at all?"

It felt as if he already knew me. I responded, "To an extent. I've seen where I was and where I am now, and it's like, man, this is an act of God. But when I was diagnosed, it was hard to swallow."

Smiling and barely containing my excitement that I was talking to an MLB player, I went into the living room where my parents were and told them.

Dad said, "Someone is fooling you, pretending to be him."

I told Desi that because of my Ma-Ma, I was a Braves fan. I told him that Chipper Jones was my favorite player and that I wanted to get to a game because it was his last season before he retired.

He replied, "Yeah, do that. I'll leave you tickets."

I ran into the living room again to tell my parents, but once again, Dad said someone was playing me good. But he eventually believed me—somewhat.

At the end of our conversation, Desi said, "You're an inspiration to me, man. I would love to talk to you more about your faith and NF2 if you're up to it."

I told him I was absolutely open to talk with him about both.

My parents agreed that we could go to the game, so we booked a hotel near the stadium in Atlanta. When we got there, we gave the will-call window my name, but they told me there were no tickets for me. I looked at my dad, and he just shook his head, convinced that I'd been played by some guy pretending to be Ian Desmond.

Then they told us to go around the stadium to the visitors/media gate. When we got there, they told us that the tickets had not arrived yet. It was about 104 degrees on the heat index, and we waited on the street curb in the shade, pouring sweat. Twenty minutes passed, and we tried making small talk with another player's family. Finally, my dad looked at me and said, "If you made us come down here without us having tickets . . ."

Then the window blinds of the ticket booth opened. We went up and gave my name as well as Desi's. There were three tickets to see the game, and Desi had even put us in the shade! It was a great game, but the Nationals lost to the Braves.

We got to meet Desi in the tunnel afterward. I was on Twitter telling him we were there and to take his time. About 20 minutes later, I received a message from him saying, "The interviews are taking forever." About 10 minutes after that, he showed up to talk to us. He asked about NF, and my parents began telling him about it.

By this time, we had been talking on Twitter for a few weeks, so I felt comfortable around him. I had a tumor in the palm of my left hand, and my mom showed it to him. He asked me if it hurt and if he could touch it. I told him no, it didn't hurt and yes, he could touch it. I lifted my hand and turned it over for him to feel it. He extended his hand to touch the tumor, but I pulled my hand back. "Ah!" I yelled, and he pulled back, his mouth and eyes wide open.

I laughed. "I'm just kidding," I said. "Do you want to touch it?"

He quickly shook his head no. We still laugh about it to this day. He said he told some teammates, and they laughed but said it was "messed up."

Later my parents asked me why I had teased him like that. I told them that I really didn't know. "It just happened," I said. "I was just comfortable around him and thought I could be myself."

After talking to Desi a bit longer, we found out what had taken him so long. He pulled out a ball signed by Chipper Jones that said, "God bless and Good luck!"

I made sure to get a picture with him and a couple of autographs.

Desi later told a reporter about the ordeal: "I had never met anyone with tumors, I was like, 'Oh man, what did you just do?' . . . That's when I knew this kid was cool."

On July 4, 2012, God gave us another special gift: Keylen "Keybug" Rice was born. I had gone to school with his parents, played sports with his dad, and gone to church with his mom and her family, so we knew the family pretty well.

As I lay in my bed sleeping on July 4, 2012, I had no idea how much my life was going to change that day. At 5:25 that morning little Keylen Rice was born, and the world became a better place—not only for me and my family but also for everyone who has the privilege of knowing him.

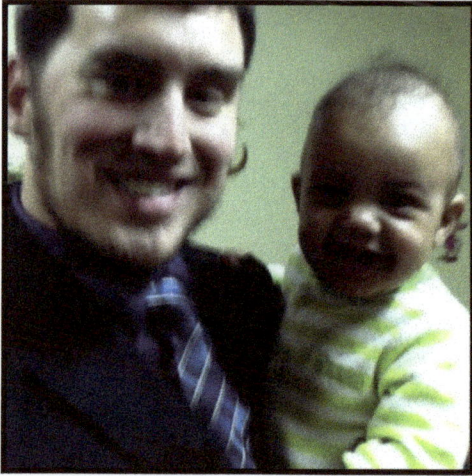

I first saw Keybug at church. He was a long, skinny baby. I really wanted to hold him but was scared I might break him. When I eventually got up the nerve, he captured my heart.

Keybug's mom, older brother, and extended family had attended my church for as long as I could remember. My mom was in charge of the nursery at church and knew that Keybug's mom was a single mom who had to work, so I wasn't too surprised when Mom offered to help by keeping Keybug on the weekends. My family quickly fell in love with him, and he really loved my mom. He became a very important part of our lives. We kept him almost every weekend—and still do.

Every Sunday morning after Sunday school, I'd go to the nursery to see him. I couldn't help but kiss him on the head or cheek.

He had a toy monkey he loved a lot. At that point I could still walk and talk clearly, so when he started standing up, I'd take him to my parents' bed and hold his hands while he jumped. I'd sing, "One little monkey jumping on the bed; one fell off and bumped his head."

One night, when Keybug's mom came to take him home, she held her hands out to Keybug, but he wouldn't leave my mom. He even drew back from her, to which she said, "You better come here. I gave birth to you!"

Keybug's dad had a cousin who played football for the University of South Carolina, so Keybug often came over wearing a Gamecock outfit. I told him that he's the only way I'd touch a Gamecock outfit.

At that time, I had begun to forget things and struggled to stay focused. When I told my mom, she said she thought it was called "chemo brain."

She had me see a psychologist who asked me if I had suicidal thoughts, and I told him no.

Now, more than ever, I sometimes let thoughts get to me. I don't have a lot to do to keep my mind busy, so it often wanders. The mind is very powerful. If you think negatively, it can have a major impact on your life.

"As water reflects the face, so one's life reflects the heart" (Prov. 27:19). That word *heart* refers to the inner man or intellect: mind, knowledge, thinking, reflection, memory. It's said that you are what you eat, and I believe it's safe to say you are what you think. If you fill your body with junk food, you'll perform like junk. If you fill your mind with negative thoughts, it'll soon show in your life. You can get depressed and do yourself and those around you serious damage.

I try to limit my contact with pessimistic people. I talk to them and try to help them through whatever it is they're going through, but if they're always negative about things, I'll distance myself. Attitudes are infectious, and I don't want to catch something else that can do me damage. Have this attitude: "This is where I am. I may not like or understand it, but I trust God to work this out for my good."

Is your attitude something others want to catch?

"The problem is not the problem; the problem is your attitude about the problem,"[1] as Captain Jack Sparrow said in *The Pirates of the Caribbean*.

Finally, the psychologist gave me IQ tests. Thankfully, I scored in the "above average" range for my age! I had no further excuse for why I was so

---

1. *The Pirates of the Caribbean*, directed by Gore Verbinski, (Burbank, CA: Walt Disney Pictures, 2003).

forgetful. At that point, I would have forgotten my own head if it weren't part of my body.

Prior to my elk hunt, the ODF had sent me on an alligator hunt in Georgetown, South Carolina. My dad and I drove to the Kinloch Plantation. Ted Turner, who owned Turner Broadcasting System (TBS) and Turner Field, former home of the Atlanta Braves, used to own the plantation.

The first afternoon, my dad, the plantation workers, and I rode around looking for our prey, and we spotted a nine-foot gator. Gators usually stay in the water, so the target area is very small. You have to shoot them behind the eyes or on the back of the head, which is the only part of the gator that is visible above water. I was 40 yards away, and it took me three shots before I finally nailed it. My dad said that he was amazed it didn't swim off after I'd missed the first two times!

The plantation manager, Brad Jones, also known as OBJ, and I became good friends after that.

The elk hunt was a few weeks later. My parents and I flew to Utah and landed at Salt Lake City International Airport. Once we claimed our luggage, we were told that a Department of Natural Resources (DNR) officer would greet us and take us to the Johnson Mountain Ranch where the hunt would be.

He was standing there holding a makeshift sign. I felt like a superstar!

After we made small talk to get acquainted, my dad rented a car. He and my mom followed the officer and me to the ranch. The officer's name was Tony, and he gave me a lot of information that day. He said that the entire area had been under water at some point in history, and if you believe in a global Noah's Flood, then you know that it was. If you look at the mountains and surrounding landscape, you can see the evidence by the markings. He also told me that many towns around the area are named after books in the Book of Mormon.

We arrived at the ranch and waited for my other three guides, Gabe, Josh, and Paul, to return from scouting for the hunt. They decided I needed to have my gun sighted, so they sighted it to make a shot 100 yards or longer.

Gabe told us, "You haven't met a redneck until you've met me!" Knowing how my mom was about rednecks, I gave a faint laugh.

Then we all went inside the house that overlooked a pond. Josh laid some stuff on a table. A friend of his who owned Shed Inc. Outdoor Gear had given me a shirt, an orange hunting hat, and two stickers for my car. He then pulled out a knife that had a handle made of elk antler and a handmade leather sheath.

That night when I was taking my shower, I picked up the body wash and saw a big black spider looking at me. I screamed and jumped out of the shower. Come to find out, the owner of the house had told my parents they had spiders, but everything else was okay.

Before I went to bed that night, I inspected my bed for critters and even sprayed spider repellent around my bed.

The next morning was a cold one. We loaded the vehicles for the hunt and headed for the trail. After riding a short way, a medium-sized bull elk and two cows (females) ran out in front of us. The elk were gone by the time I got out of the vehicle.

Gabe had the microphone my teachers had used in my classes, so he could tell me when to shoot. They set Tony and me on a hill, calling or bugling. The elk didn't move as Gabe wanted, so Tony, Dad, and I moved to another spot closer to the elk. Josh called the elk, and it moved out in the opening for a shot. The elk was dark brown and standing next to trees. Gabe gave me the green light to shoot. The only problem was that my scope was on nine because they were preparing for a long shot, but I had an elk within 40 yards. Gabe was whispering over and over, "Shoot! Shoot!"

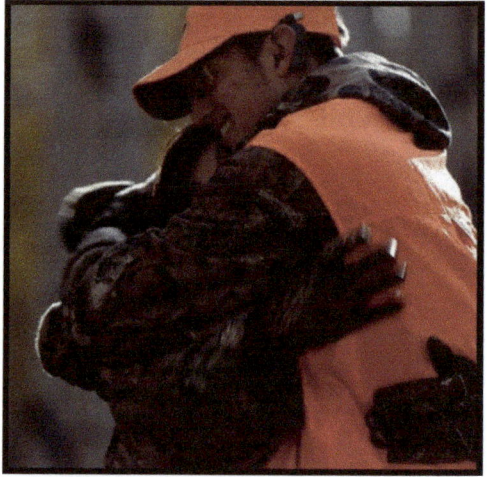

I had no idea whether I was about to shoot an elk or a tree. I closed my eyes as I pulled the trigger. Next thing I knew, I heard shouts and saw my mom running and stumbling toward me. She was crying as she hugged me.

"Are you okay?" I asked.

"These are happy tears. I'm just so happy for you!" she replied.

I had shot the elk in the neck. It had taken one step and gone down. I had shot a 6x6 elk. My guide Josh made a YouTube video and still pictures of my hunt: "Ethan's 2012 Utah Elk Hunt."

Before we left the ranch a few days later, Officer Tony Wood gave me his badge. Josh also gave me the ivory from my elk.

Around that time, Sam Kelly asked me if I'd be interested in speaking to the Chapman High School football team, and I agreed.

After we set the details, the coach said he wanted me to give a five- to ten-minute pregame devotion. I felt led to speak on Paul and Silas in jail. For those who aren't familiar with the story in Acts 16:25–31, Paul and Silas are thrown into prison because Paul rebuked a spirit from a girl who brought her owners a lot of money by fortune-telling. When her owners realized that their way of making money was gone, they dragged Paul and Silas before the magistrates of the city.

They ordered Paul and Silas to be beaten and thrown into prison. So, they put Paul and Silas in the inner prison and locked their feet in stocks. Around midnight, Paul and Silas were praying and singing praises to God as the other prisoners listened on. Then a great earthquake shook the foundations of the prison, opening all the prison doors and loosening all the chains that bound the prisoners.

Right here, I'm sure many people will tell you that praising God more will make your troubles disappear. I can tell you that this is simply not true. What is true is that when you're in "prison," the "prisoners" are watching and listening to you, especially if you are a Christian. Paul and Silas didn't make a run for it. When the jailor saw them still there, he asked Paul and Silas what he must do to be saved.

Matthew Henry, a seventeenth-century Bible commentator, says that Satan will distract us when we are serving God, seeking to upset us and stir our emotions when we should be controlled.[2]

Recently, I was leaving the gym in my wheelchair when a woman told me that if I had loved Jesus more, I wouldn't be in my wheelchair. I told some friends about it. One of them got really angry and said she couldn't believe someone had said that to me. She said that she believed in God because of me—because she has seen the miracles that He has done in my life. "You're a miracle!" she said.

In a 2013 interview for Unashamed Athletes, Desi said, "Ethan's faith absolutely strengthened me to know fully that God has a plan for us, to be happy, not scared, nervous, or anxious. When times get hard in life, baseball, or whatever situation, have faith in God and his plan, and you can find contentment. Ethan defines this."

No matter what your "prison" might be, sing praises. "Prisoners" are watching and listening.

---

2. Bible Study Tools, s.v. "Matthew Henry Commentary on the Whole Bible: Acts: Acts 16" https://www.biblestudytools.com/commentaries/matthew-henry-complete/acts/16.html.

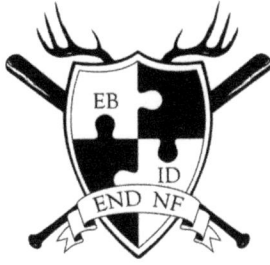

CHAPTER 8

I had to stop the Avastin chemo because I was spilling protein into my urine, an issue that could cause kidney problems. I was maintaining a 3.0 GPA in college even with the distraction of a busy schedule and having to see various doctors. With the exception of having to come off chemo, everything was going pretty well.

The Nationals were playing the Braves in April 2013, so I texted Desi to see if I could come to Atlanta to see him play. It was close to final exams, so I called it a reward for the hard work I had put in all semester. He agreed and gave a friend and me tickets and batting-practice passes so we could talk to him before the game.

My friend Harley and I ate at the Varsity, a place well known for its hamburgers. Many famous and important people have eaten there. I didn't think the hamburgers were anything special—just two small patties like any fast-food joint. To me, my dad makes a better burger.

We got to the game three hours before game time. Once we got inside the stadium, we walked down to the field. The Nationals weren't out yet, so we decided to watch the Braves' batting practice. Harley leaned over and said, "Ball on bat is really loud in person compared to TV."

He was a Braves fan, so I pointed across the field and said, "There's Freddie Freeman," a four-time All-Star.

He recognized him and said, "Those goggles make him look terrifying, don't they?"

I couldn't help but laugh at that.

A few minutes later I got a tap on the shoulder from a stadium worker who said, "That man over there wants to see you." I looked over and saw Desi sitting against the foul-ball net. I tapped my friend on the shoulder and said, "Follow me. We're going to meet Desi."

Harley was like a kid on Christmas morning; he was so excited to meet a Major League Baseball All-Star.

"Hey Desi, what's up?" I called out as we approached him.

"Nothing much. Got ready, and I'm spitting seeds now. I didn't know y'all would actually watch batting practice."

"Yeah, man," I said. "We had to do something to pass the time."

After talking to Desi a bit, I introduced my friend. "This is Harley. He's a Braves fan, so talk slow to him."

Harley reached out to shake Desi's hand, and I noticed a tattoo of the word *Family* on his opposite wrist.

I told him if he hit the Chick-fil-A cow on top of the stadium in the left outfield, I'd buy my game tickets from then on.

He smiled. "I've already hit it." Then he said he had to go hit in the cage and that he'd be back. As he was drilling the balls, Harley looked at me and said, "He better save some for the game."

A few minutes later, Desi returned to talk to us more. I noticed another tattoo peeking out of his shirt in his collarbone area. That sparked me to ask how many tattoos he had.

He replied, "I have eight. Would you get one if I got another one?"

I looked at him kind of in shock; then I looked at Harley and back to Desi. "Yeah, man! I've thought about a tattoo before," I said.

Desi remembers this story differently. He says that I didn't want to do it because I'd be too scared. "Do you know what I go through?" he says I asked him.

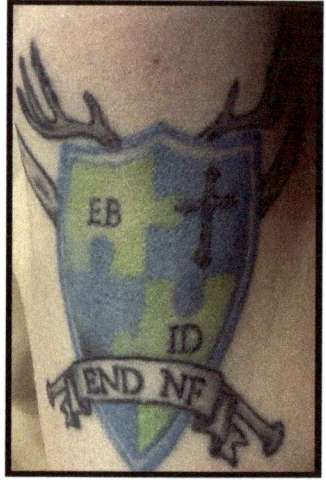

Either way, I did get one—a matching one with Desi.

He had to finish warming up, but before he left, he asked me whether I had brought a jacket. I told him I left it in the car and that I'd be fine. "You sure?" he asked. "It's going to be cold tonight." I told him, yes, I was sure. Then we shook hands, and he went off to the dugout.

I turned and started to walk away when I heard my name called. I turned around and saw Desi with a jacket. He handed it to me and took off. I held it out in front of me and read it: "Nationals 20," Desi's number. I looked at Harley and said, "You've got an authentic jersey, and I've got an authentic jacket."

Later that summer, my parents and I went to Washington, DC, for my 21st birthday. I texted Desi and told him we had been given Fan Appreciation Day tickets, which allowed fans to access the stadium, get a T-shirt, and walk on the field to see their favorite players.

Shortly after Desi and I first met, he tweeted that if I had 2,000 followers by the end of that night, he'd give away tickets to a game. I racked up lots of followers but never reached 2,000.

At the stadium, I tweeted that I was at Fan Appreciation Day. I had Twitter followers wanting to meet me and take pictures with me. I felt like a celebrity.

I texted Desi, and he told us to go down to the field. Once down there, we waited for Desi to walk by like the other players. When I saw him, I called out and waved to get him to stop by. After talking a bit, he pulled me out of the crowd. Someone called, "Hey, Desi, what about me?"

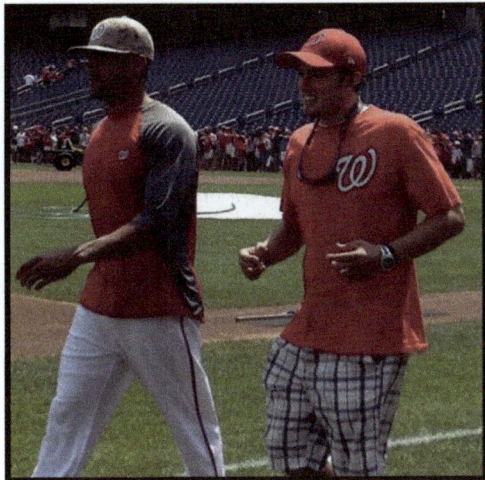

He responded, "This is my boy!"

As we were walking to the dugout, he told me that I had to help him wave to the crowd. We were shown on the big screen and met by a woman who helps with the team. "Hi, Ethan, can I get you anything? A drink?" she asked.

Desi jumped in. "He doesn't drink, right?"

I smiled at him. "Yeah, I don't drink. The medicine I'm on doesn't allow it." I wouldn't have taken a drink even if I could have.

After leaving her behind, we made our way to the dugout. A guy jumped in front of me and told me I wasn't allowed to go in there. I thought to myself, *"That worked out well!"* Then Desi said, "He's with me."

I puffed my chest up and thought to myself, *"Yeah, back off!"*

We went into the dugout, and I saw stairs leading up. Desi told me to follow him. I did as he said, not knowing where we were going. At the top, I saw someone working out. Desi called out, "Stras, you got a minute?" Stephen Strasburg, who was drafted with the very first pick in the 2009 Major League Baseball draft, came over to shake my hand. "This is my friend Ethan."

"Wait," I thought. He just called me his friend! He laughed about it that night when I told him.

"I hope that's what we are," he said.

I was someone to him, not just a random fan he pulled out of the crowd, not just Ethan, but his friend. Jesus calls us a friend (if we obey his teaching and accept him as Lord), and He no longer calls us servants. How cool is it that the same God who created the universe calls us friends? We aren't just Ethan or whatever your name may be; we are his friends!

After we talked with Stras a few minutes, Desi showed me around the clubhouse and his locker. We started to head out as Adam LaRoche and his son came in. After talking to them a bit, we headed back out once more. It was a thrilling day.

That night I got on Twitter and saw that a follower who was at the event had posted a picture of me and Desi walking back to join my parents.

We went to the game that night. Desi gave us Diamond Club tickets for seats where there was food and more throughout the game. The Nationals won the game, and as we were leaving, Mom heard someone shouting my name. It turned out to be another Twitter follower. I had my name on the back of the hat I was wearing. It's always fun to meet strangers who know you and make connections.

After the game the next day, we met Desi. I shook his hand and gave him a bro hug. When I hugged Desi, I noticed he was warm, so I asked, "Did you just shower?"

"Yeah, do I smell good?" he answered.

Not sure how to answer, I laughingly said, "Yeah, man."

We met Desi's wife, Chelsey, and two of their sons.

After the Washington trip, I volunteered at a camp. The night before the camp started, I was given the option to stay at camp or go out to a bar with some other staffers. I told one guy that I would not drink but wanted to go. He told me that was fine and that I was more than welcome to come.

Once inside, everyone but me ordered their favorite beverage. We sat and talked for a solid two hours or more.

A lot of times the same people who say that only God can judge them are the ones who judge me for being a Christian. They seem to think I will take their fun away, making them skittish to ask me to do things or invite me to places. That couldn't be further from the truth as the staffers found out that night. I may not do what others do, but I'm still a human too.

After the camp, my balance decreased every day. A new semester was starting, and doctors said that I was looking at a possible surgery in December. I had changed my major to graphic design. I loved sitting behind a computer and designing photos. I was still unsure of what I wanted to do, so Dad talked to Sam Kelly, who gave me a job working in the warehouse at Sam Group. Sam allowed me to meet Tim Tebow by buying a table for an event. One of the classes required for my new major was kicking my rear end; I'd come home and put my nose in the textbook for hours.

On fall break, Mom, Dad, and I took Keybug to the beach. It was a great getaway from the hassle of school, balance issues, and a possible surgery in December. That trip to the beach helped me, but I was still very stressed about school. Having Keybug with us helped a lot. It was his first trip to the beach, and he was a pleasure to watch. For some reason, he loved to eat the sand. But I guess most kids do that. We took Keybug to Magic Kingdom and let him do a lot of the rides; he loved them. Seeing him smile made me smile.

After we got back from the beach, we were invited to hunt deer at a farm that raises big deer. On the morning of the first day in the field, one of the hunters tapped me on the knee. On the left, there were two does—female deer—so I felt good about my chances of getting a buck. Ten minutes later, I was about half-asleep when I felt a rush of heavy taps on my leg. There was a huge buck about 80 yards out. It stopped in front of a pine tree, got up on his back legs, locked its antlers with a limb, and gave me a broadside shot. My companion gave me a thumbs-up to pull the trigger.

I looked into the scope, found the deer, took a deep breath in, and slowly exhaled as I squeezed the trigger. I saw a red flash in the scope as the bullet exploded out of the barrel. The deer kicked as if I'd hit it but then it took off in a sprint. "You missed him!" my partner said.

Turns out, my dad unintentionally sabotaged me. He can be cheap, and before the hunt, he sighted my gun with cheap bullets. When we got to the farm after the morning miss, a person shot my gun with the bullets I'd been using and said the gun was way off.

My hunting partner set up an afternoon hunt for which I was wide awake. He told me that he was going to "corn 'em up." After we had been sitting for about 30 to 40 minutes, five bucks walked out and started eating the corn. I was thrilled! They were 40 yards away and set up for an easy shot.

But just then, a bug got caught in my throat. I started coughing, and the deer jerked up to see what was going on. My partner told me that they hadn't seen us, but he wouldn't let me pull the trigger yet. Then the deer looked up to the right and dashed off. I was bummed. Deer were right there in front of us, and I had to let them go. A few minutes later, a light tap on my leg revealed there was a big deer about 80 yards off. I slowly adjusted to shoot, took a deep breath, locked eyes firmly on the deer, and pulled the trigger.

"You got him!" My hunting partner was thrilled, and so was I.

After the trip, my balance was much worse, especially on uneven ground. My dad thought my lack of balance came from looking at my phone too much. We had slippery hardwood floors at home, and Dad said I fell because I was looking at my phone instead of where I was going.

I was also struggling with a class. Our final project was to design a webpage, and I couldn't complete it. The day the project was due, I had tears in my eyes. I told the class that I didn't know how to do the assignment; my balance was worsening, and I was facing brain surgery in a few weeks. The teacher took me outside and told me not to worry about the assignment, that he'd take care of it.

I stayed in the hospital the night before my surgery, and we FaceTimed Keybug and his mom. He loved talking to me as much as I loved talking to him.

On the day of my surgery, I had to wear a red surgery hat. I FaceTimed Desi and told him the difference between him in red (his team color) and me in red was that I made it look good!

That surgery at Duke took nine hours, and I spent a day in intensive care. Then I was moved to a regular room. I wasn't eating, so they

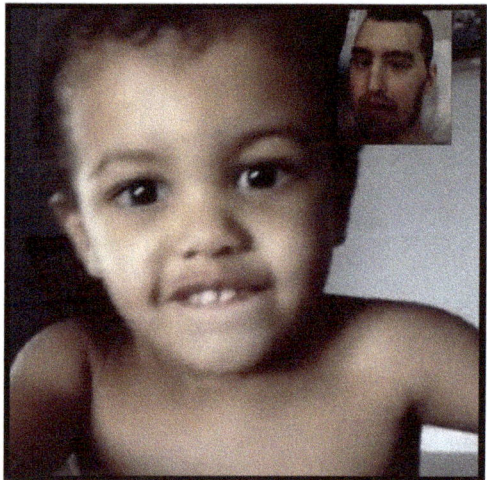

scheduled me to have a temporary feeding tube in my nose. I used that for a few days.

One night, my parents took me out of my room so I could see the hospital. I was already having problems with the feeding tube because I often burped the "food" they gave me. While we were in the pediatric part of the hospital, I sneezed, and the tube almost came out. I knew I needed it, so when it came out and was choking me, I tried to let it go. But it kept making me gag, so I decided to pull it out.

My parents gasped when it happened. "You need that!" Mom said. We immediately went back to the room to tell the nurse what had happened. She said it was okay because the tube was probably already coming out since I had been tasting the "food" they were giving me. I started eating solid food so that the doctors at Duke would let me go home. I had to go straight to a rehab hospital, but at least I was back in South Carolina.

At the rehab hospital, Sam Kelly and Jamal came by with a monetary gift and a card that said, "We love you, but Jesus loves you more."

The next day, Keybug came, and was I happy to see him! That little boy saw me and threw his arms around my neck! He loves me no matter what.

The world would be better off if there were more Keybugs!

Since one of my friends goes to church with Matthew Le-Croy's family, she convinced him and his wife to visit me in 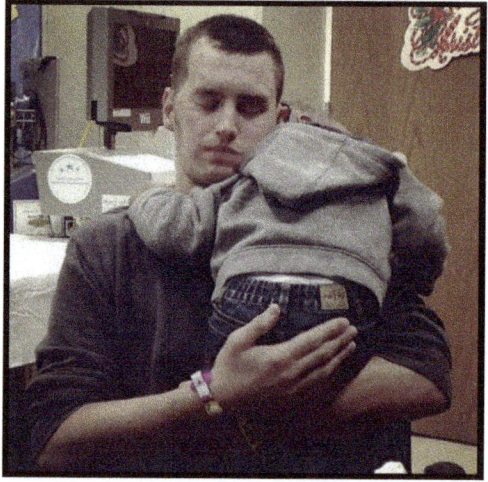 the rehab hospital. Matthew LeCroy should be a familiar name to Clemson baseball fans: he played for Clemson and then was drafted in the first round. I have one of his baseball cards from his days in the big league. At that time LeCroy was the bullpen coach for the Nationals, and he knew Desi. We bonded over our connections with Desi and took a picture to send to him.

Desi asked, "What is he doing there?"

I showed his text to my dad, who told me to tell Desi that LeCroy was in the area scouting shortstop talent (Desi was drafted as a shortstop before leaving the Nationals).

"Ha!" Desi replied. "He wouldn't know what talent was if he saw it. He'd know pizza if he saw it though."

I laughed and responded, "You better watch it; he may tell Coach to make you run more."

"He wouldn't tattle on me; we go way back! Don't trade that Desmond jersey in for a LeCroy one. I knew you first!"

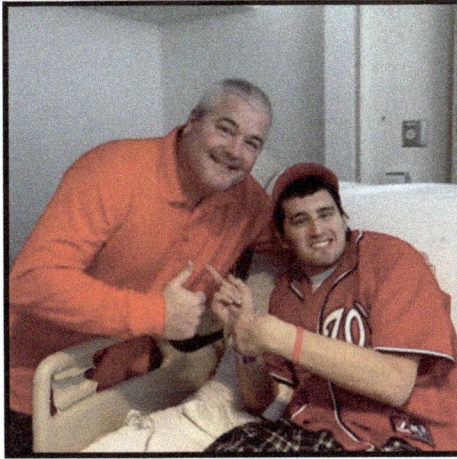

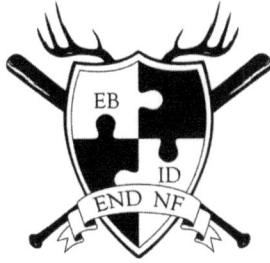

CHAPTER 9

My doctors at Duke believed that another surgery was my next best option. I was reluctant because it would leave me completely deaf, because the cochlear implant had been inserted through the tumor, which was now causing problems.

It devastated me to think about deafness. I wrestled with God over and over again. What would I do if the fire alarm went off and I couldn't hear it? I'd never hear my parents' voices again, birds, music—anything. Throughout my life, I had been deeply touched by music, and it was especially important to me during all my surgeries and therapies. I couldn't bear to think that soon I wouldn't be hearing those songs anymore. One of my favorites was "Who I Am Hates Who I've Been" by Relient K.

One day, my pastor stopped by to visit and brought the youth pastor's guitar. After we talked for a while, he picked up the guitar and said, "I'm really not very good at this, but I'll give it a try." Then he sang the old hymn "Have Thine Own Way, Lord." There's a line in that song that stood out to me: "Thou art the potter, I am the clay. Mold me and make me after thy will." Hearing those words, I couldn't help but think that I just wanted to be better. To me, *better* meant walking by myself, hearing, and speaking clearly.

In addition to not being able to hear my music, I worried about how being deaf would affect my relationships with other people.

I believe God answered me through my mom: "If someone really loves you, they won't mind at all!"

I often asked my parents whether I had to do the surgery and whether there were other options.

There were none.

"Look, Ethan," they said, "we hate this just as much as you do, but it's your hearing or your life. We'd much rather it be your hearing. You're our only son."

Then my mom took me in her arms and rocked me.

Since everything during this tough time seemed to stress me out, my parents and I took a weekend trip to Georgia to get my mind off things back home. It didn't work. When they saw that I was still depressed, they said, "We love you, Ethan. We would take this from you if we could."

"You know I wouldn't let you," I said. "Nobody deserves to have to deal with this."

In Matthew 26:39, Jesus had taken His disciples to the Garden of Gethsemane to pray with Him. "Going a little farther, he fell with his face to the ground and prayed, 'My Father, if it is possible, may this cup be taken from me. Yet not as I will, but as you will.'"

The Bible says that in his anguish, Jesus sweated blood. That actually can happen. It's a known medical condition called hematidrosis, which happens on rare occasions and is associated with high psychological stress. Severe anxiety releases chemicals that break down the capillaries in the sweat glands. As a result, a small amount of blood bleeds into those glands and comes out in the sweat.

Jesus was fully God, but He also was fully man. It wasn't easy for Him, but He surrendered to His

Father's will. Likewise, this wasn't easy for me, but, like Jesus, I wanted God's will to be done.

"Why, my soul, are you downcast? Why so disturbed within me? Put your hope in God, for I will yet praise him, my Savior and my God" (Ps. 42:5).

My mom often told me that God had not brought me this far to abandon me.

Before my surgery, I messaged an old friend on Facebook to see whether she wanted to see a movie with me. We had been friends for a long time, so I didn't hesitate to ask her whether it'd be weird for my parents to take me.

"It'll only be weird if you make it weird," she replied.

It was a huge deal to me that I was in a wheelchair and couldn't drive, but I tried to play it off when I met her there. I bought our tickets, and she helped push me around when I struggled to get rolling. Everything seemed to be going well—at least in my mind.

Toward the end of the movie, *The Fault in Our Stars*, the main character is in a wheelchair, and his girlfriend pushes him around. Not knowing the story, I thought to myself, *"Oh this is great!"* Then, in the next scene, his girlfriend is by herself with the wheelchair because the boyfriend had died. Not the most uplifting ending for a guy like me to watch!

The next weekend, my parents were grilling hamburgers. I asked my friend whether she would like to come over, and she agreed. But when I texted back to confirm, she said her mom wouldn't let her come.

I asked her to let me talk to her mom, but she wouldn't. After I persisted, she finally told me the truth: "I think it's best we stay friends."

Her mom never had said she couldn't come.

I was hurt that she felt the need to lie about it. She told me we'd "stay friends," but we never talked again. Whenever I messaged her, she would ignore me.

I have often tried to find some type of relationship on my own, only to have it sputter and end quickly. People have heard about me from school, television, radio, newspaper interviews, family, or peers. They want to meet me, but they don't want to get too close.

I often feel left out in public because no one uses or knows sign language well. People try to talk to me, but if I'm alone, it usually doesn't go well. I don't want to seem rude by being on my phone, but my phone is how I communicate. I have been told to text what I want to say, but then people don't realize I'm trying to text messages to them. They think I'm just texting and lose patience and walk away. It can be difficult and very disappointing.

My parents and I took a beginner sign language course, so we know a bit. But my parents still prefer to text me because ASL is very difficult. I prayed for a friend who wasn't family because family should always love you and stick with you no matter what.

When May 2014 rolled around, Desi announced his "End NF" campaign. (May is not only NF Awareness Month, but it's also my birthday month.) After making his campaign public, the stories started to pop up. One story was published by Patrick Reddington on federalbaseball.com. "My goal is to just get this out," Desi said in the article. "I want to spread the word about this thing and hopefully it can rally some people behind us." He explained his drive to raise awareness of NF, something so few people know anything about. "The goal of the Indiegogo campaign is to raise money for the Children's Tumor Foundation and awareness of the impact NF has on more than two million people worldwide.[3]

The original goal for the campaign was $10,000, but in less than a week of going public, Desi and those helping him passed that and set sights on $20,000.

---

3. Patrick Reddington, "Nationals' SS Ian Desmond, #steak and the Campaign to #EndNF" SBNation Federal Baseball, May 7, 2014, https://www.federalbaseball.com/2014/5/7/5689988/nationals-ss-ian-desmond-on-steak-and-the-campaign-to-endnf.

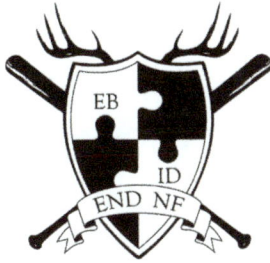

CHAPTER 10

As May was ending, my parents, aunt, and cousin invited our new associate pastor and his wife to supper at Red Lobster for my 22nd birthday. Everyone tried to make it a fun evening, but I couldn't help but think it would be the last birthday I'd be able to hear. The thought was on my mind almost constantly.

Earlier, my mom had decided to get a tattoo. That really surprised me because she isn't one to tolerate pain well. As soon as she expects the slightest pain, she goes to the medicine cabinet.

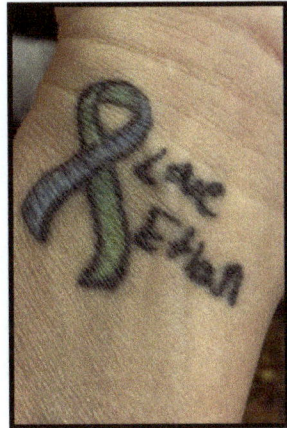

She decided to get an NF ribbon that has "Love Ethan" in my handwriting inked on her wrist. They say love will make you do crazy things, and this was certainly crazy to me! I guess she will do anything for me. She made me go with her to hold her hand.

After we ate, Mom asked the new pastor and his wife what they thought of tattoos and showed her ink off.

"It's for Ethan; that's sweet!" was all they said.

By the end of May, Desi's End NF campaign had reached $30,000. Desi added $16,000 of his own money after promising $1,000 for each run that he batted in.

In early June, the Nationals were on a road series that took them to San Francisco and St. Louis. While on the road, Desi got his matching NF tattoo as promised. He sent me a picture of it and asked what I thought.

"Looks great!" I texted back.

It turned out to be a bigger deal than either of us expected. His fans noticed the tattoo, and a story by Scott Allen appeared in the *Washington Post*.[4]

---

4. Scott Allen, "The Story Behind Ian Desmond's 'End NF' Tattoo Is Incredible" *Washington Post*, June 18, 2014, https://www.washingtonpost.com/news/dc-sports-bog/wp/2014/06/18/the-story-behind-ian-desmonds-end-nf-tattoo-is-incredible/

For my birthday gift, Mom texted Desi and asked whether he would leave tickets for us to see a game. He said yes, so we flew to DC. For the home-stand, the team magazine ran a story on Desi and me titled "A Means to an End."

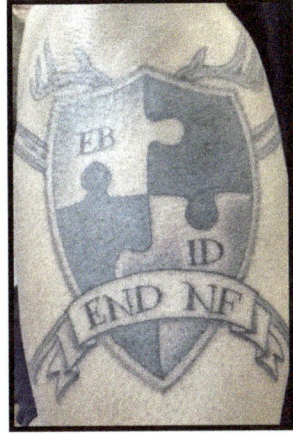

The day we headed to the game was Military Appreciation Day at the ballpark, and during batting practice, I caught a group of Navy SEALs staring at me, then back at the magazine. A member of the group came over and asked whether that was me in the magazine and whether they could have a picture. Before I could say anything, Mom answered for me: "He'd love to!"

When I had attended a game the previous year, I had been able to walk. This time I was confined to a wheelchair. Back at the hotel, Desi texted that I'd better get my legs in gear because he wasn't pushing me. He followed that by texting, "I'm just kidding. I'll push you, but we may have to pop a few wheelies."

At that time, Desi and his wife were expecting a son. He liked Florida State University and supported a win against Clemson (FSU won a national championship). Before we left for home, we gave him a gift: a baby-sized Clemson shirt.

Jimbo Redden, who had done Mom's and my tattoos, and his wife, Jennifer, invited me to Jimbo's birthday celebration in Clemson, a party that would include some Clemson football players.

I messed my clothes up by accident on the way and got so frustrated that I told Mom to forget about going. She's stubborn and wants me happy at whatever cost, so we stopped to get a change of clothes at Walmart along the way.

I was putting the shorts on when I noticed they were two sizes too big. That was all they had, and we had no time to spare because we were already late.

As we pulled up and started to get out of the car, my shorts fell to my ankles. If that wasn't embarrassing enough, two college students were walking by. They laughed (I could still hear at the time), but I sure didn't. Mom apologized, and we made our way into the place to meet Jimbo and company. We had a great night and made some new friends in spite of it all.

Before we headed to Duke for my surgery, the Outdoor Dream Foundation invited me out to fish near the beach. After fishing a bit, we got cleaned up and went out to eat. We made a stop at a public beach spot so I could hear the ocean and the seagulls squawking one last time. It was a nice little getaway before heading up to Duke.

At Duke, the night before my surgery, I sat in my hospital bed listening to the old hymn "What a Friend We Have in Jesus" for the last time. I tried talking to Dad, but I couldn't resist the song. It gave me such peace, even knowing I would be deaf the next day. That night would have seemed like forever, but thankfully, I got some sleep. I also stared at the ceiling a lot.

The night before my surgery, three familiar faces came into my room: my great-aunt and great-uncle and the associate pastor. I honestly wasn't expecting any visitors because Duke is a long way from home. I tried to hear all the *I love you*s I could from my parents. I wanted to memorize those sounds. Mom actually got in bed with me while I waited the next morning.

The surgery successfully debulked the tumor, they thought, and took my hearing. I was discharged in a few days but had to go straight to a rehab hospital. For about a week, I worked on balance, strength, coordination, and sign language. I started each day at eight in the morning and ended around four that afternoon.

I told Desi that I was getting cheesecake every meal.

He answered, "Cheesecake and naps? Sounds like a vacation!"

"Work hard, nap hard, Desi!" I replied.

One night, I was eating supper with Mom when we noticed I was struggling to keep food and liquid in my mouth. Mom rushed me back to the floor and told the nurses. As soon as I was in bed, they called the stroke team and rushed me to the night doctor. Mom wasn't there, and it was so late that there was no translator to help me communicate.

The doctor became frustrated because I couldn't understand him. I shouted to the nurse, "I do not like that doctor! He makes me feel stupid, and I'm not!" The doctor got so frustrated he threw his hands up and left.

Sometimes, people are unkind to deaf people. When you meet someone from a foreign country, do you assume that person is stupid? No. At least, you shouldn't. They speak a different language, but chances are they are as smart or smarter than you. It's the same with people who are deaf.

I eventually saw a new doctor. I liked this one better because he wrote what he wanted to say to me. He said my problem was most likely Bell's palsy, which causes sudden, temporary weakness in your facial muscles. It made half my face appear to droop, my smile become one-sided, and my eye on that side stay half-closed.

I was discharged from the hospital for a month, but then I was back at Duke for another surgery because they didn't get as much of the tumor as they needed to get the first time.

Before the surgery, Mom, Dad, and I took Keybug to Atlanta to meet Desi. Keybug was so excited about the trip. Our room was connected to the courtyard by a sliding glass door, and my parents decided to let him burn some energy before the game. After he played, my parents took him back to the room while they got ready. He was running around in his diaper, yelling, "Baseball!" He was so hyped that he didn't see the glass door and ran right into it and fell backward. He didn't know what hit him! I couldn't help but laugh.

At the game, we introduced Keybug. When Desi held out his hands, Keybug didn't hesitate to go to him. Desi took him off a short distance to play with him and toss a baseball. We made a video of them, and it's probably my favorite thing to watch.

It was a great game, and Keybug made it even better. If I happened to take my eyes off the field, he would tap my arm and point to the field. I guess he didn't want me to miss anything!

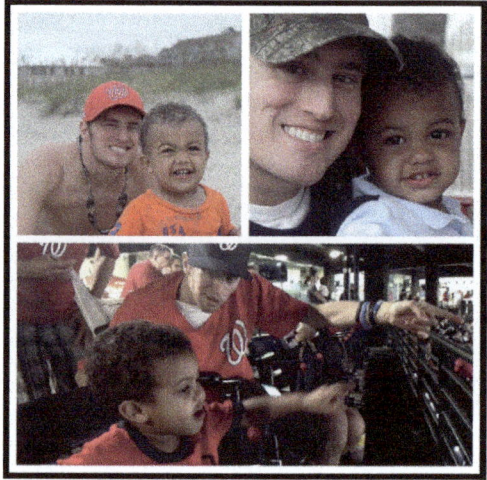

My mom's office made me a shirt with my name on the front and a picture of Desi's and my tattoo on the back.

My favorite Bible verse, Psalm 23:4, was underneath the picture: "Even though I walk through the darkest valley, I will fear no evil, for you are with me; your rod and your staff, they comfort me."

My mom took a picture of the shirt and uploaded it to Facebook. It wasn't long until the comments "I want one" or "How can I get one?" started coming in. We sold over 150 shirts. We couldn't believe people actually wanted them!

I traveled to Duke with Mom and a friend who worked for the Greenville hospital. She went with us to help me communicate better with the doctor before my next surgery.

Having my friend there was a blessing and a curse as well. She was excellent at ASL, so when the interpreter for the hospital got there, I was grateful to have her. But a few days later, I became bitter toward her. I guess I was actually bitter about my situation, wishing I was better—not deaf, in ICU, in a wheelchair, in the hospital. I'm sure my attitude made her job awful. Eventually, she even stopped coming into the room.

One night, as I was in the room watching Monday Night Football, she sat out in the hall. I remember thinking, *"You can come in here."* When she finally did and tried to make small talk, I shut her out.

I wish I could go back and redo it, because now I'd have a better attitude toward her. Just like with the nurse I called Beth after my surgery years before, I was scared. Fear and pain sometimes make it hard to be a nice person.

The moral is that no matter how tough, trying, or frustrating your situation is, always be nice to others. They're just doing their job.

One day, I was sitting in my hospital bed playing hangman with my friend while my mom was busy cleaning the room—I mean really cleaning! She even scrubbed the bathroom with Pine-Sol! I thought nothing of it because whenever we go anywhere, one of the first things she does is clean.

I should have suspected something was going to happen because she was wearing a Nationals shirt, but I figured it was just a shirt she brought along.

My friend's eyes darted around the room looking for a word so we could play. She found something and drew nine short lines. I started with vowels.

I correctly guessed two *a*'s, *i*, and *o*. Then I asked if there were any *n*'s, and she wrote in two. *N-a-i-o-n-a*. I smiled at her and guessed the word: *Nationals*. Then she and my mom told me to look at the doorway. A tall figure was there—Desi!

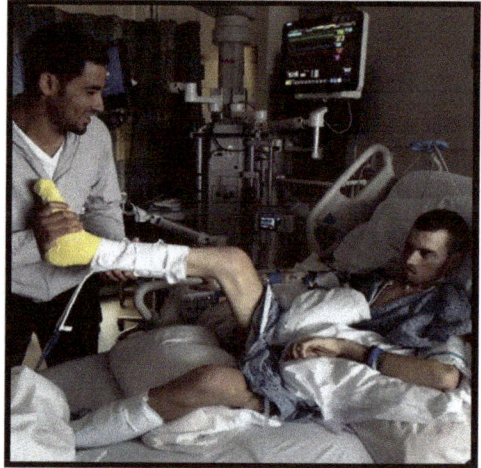

I smiled from ear to ear. "Why are you in North Carolina instead of Washington, DC?"

"I'm just out flying," he responded with a grin.

We sat and talked a while. I couldn't believe that someone who needed a plane to get here actually came to see me. I didn't ask for it. He came on his own. He helped me stretch my legs and work them. Before he left, he hugged me, which I wasn't expecting.

When he was gone, I asked my friend whether she knew that Desi was going to show up. She said no. Desi and Mom had planned the whole thing.

Later, Mom showed me a picture on her phone. Desi had taken a selfie in a Clemson hat. I guess you can teach an old dog new tricks! His friendship was—and still is—such a comfort. He's more than a friend; he's my brother. Whenever I need advice, I go to him. I know he won't tell me what I want to hear, but what I need to hear.

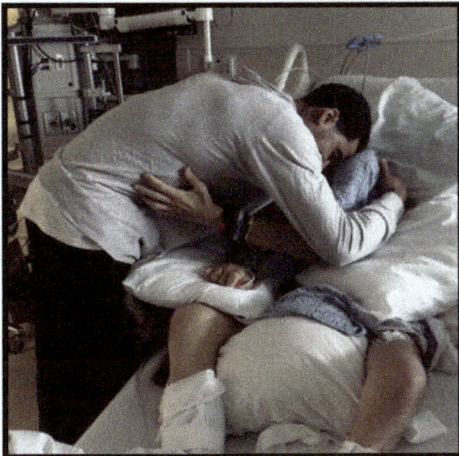

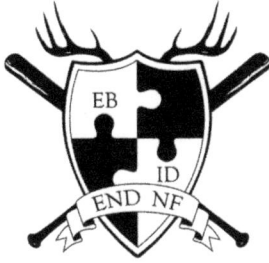

CHAPTER 11

I don't remember much about what happened after Desi came to see me at Duke. That's probably because I was highly medicated and physically traumatized. After a few weeks, they flew me to the hospital in Greenville.

I had developed a bedsore at Duke, something pretty common for a bedridden patient. It started small, but by Christmas it had grown to the size of a small grapefruit. I also developed trouble breathing. I couldn't keep my airway open, especially if I tried to tilt my head back.

The doctor told me I needed a tracheotomy, a surgical procedure during which a doctor cuts an incision on the outside of the neck and opens a direct airway through the trachea (windpipe). The resulting stoma (hole) can serve independently as an airway or as a site for a tracheal tube or tracheostomy tube to be inserted; this tube allows a person to breathe without the use of the nose or mouth. I was grateful to have it because it actually kept me alive.

I wasn't drinking enough fluid, and I had lost so much weight from not eating. I was so uncoordinated that I had to wear a big bib. It was humiliating. Sometimes, I'd eat a little just to satisfy my parents and therapist and then say I was full. During those months, I lost almost 100 pounds.

The doctors decided to insert a feeding tube, requiring another painful surgery. I was still recovering from the bedsore, yet for the procedure they had me lie flat on a hard surface. I was very uncomfortable, and the typical anesthetic didn't work. I could feel them cutting me.

Afterward, I couldn't leave the hospital, so my parents had to find someone to cut my hair. The stylist who was going to cut it came while a friend of mine who worked at the hospital was visiting me. I don't know what method they were using, but I thought they had strands of my hair pulled up in suction tubes. I was curious to know what was going on, so I reached my hand up there only to have it slapped. After a few more slaps on the wrist, I locked eyes with my friend and signed, "That person is mean!" She laughed and shook her head yes!

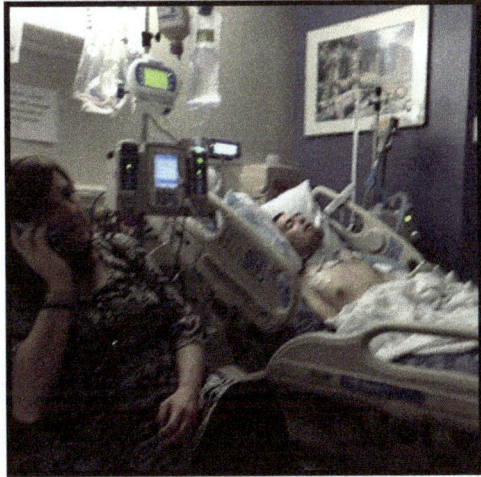

I really wanted to be home for Christmas and often asked my parents whether they thought I would be. There was no way to know, but they hoped I would be.

My dad does lawn care as a second job, so it was easier for Mom to stay at the hospital with me at night during the week. Her job is 15 minutes from the hospital, and she has the option to work from home or wherever she may be. If my dad stayed with me, he would have to leave his lawn care equipment overnight in the hospital parking lot.

One day, my extended family came to visit, and I didn't know why. I asked my parents why everyone was there, and they told me that it was Christmas. That made me very sad because that wasn't how I wanted my Christmas to be.

After the holidays, my doctor from Duke said he wanted to do shunt surgery. A shunt is a hollow tube surgically placed in the brain (or occasionally in the spine) to help drain cerebrospinal fluid to relieve pressure and redirect the fluid to another location in the body where it can be reabsorbed. They wanted mine to drain into my stomach.

My doctor said the surgery "should make everything better." I didn't know what he meant by that, but all I was concerned about was walking by myself again. When I asked my mom whether the surgery would make me walk again, she just shrugged.

The flight to Duke was very uncomfortable because of the bedsore, which still hadn't healed, and I wasn't allowed to turn on my side. I still had my IV in, so the nurse who was with me gave me pain medicine as often as I could have it.

The shunt surgery was a success, and my dad surprised me by driving up to Duke. The stay wasn't bad at all. The room was big, and my parents had a nice spot to sleep. And there were two TVs! I had a seizure in my sleep during my stay at Duke, and the doctor said it was probably from the surgery.

I've been blessed to have good nurses through the years, but one nurse really stood out during this particular stay at Duke. I wish I had gotten her name. She was about my age, and she not only did her job, but she also tried to communicate with me. At the end of her shift, she'd pull up a chair beside my bed and sit there typing on my phone, thanking me for letting her take care of me.

After a few days, I was headed back to Greenville. The flight back was as bad as the flight to Duke because of that horrendous bedsore. When I got back to Greenville, the entire Clemson basketball team visited me. My hospital room was really crowded that day!

Then they moved me to another hospital for rehabilitation. After a few weeks, the doctor said, "We really think you should do colostomy surgery. We think it will speed up the bedsore healing. You don't have to do it. Just think about it and let us know."

A colostomy brings one end of the large intestine out through an opening (stoma) made in the abdominal wall. Stools moving through the intestine drain through the stoma into a bag attached to the abdomen. I really didn't want to do the surgery, but I wanted the sore to heal. Ma-Ma had sores and open wounds on the backs of her legs that wouldn't heal, and I often asked Mom if I would be like her.

After talking it over with my parents, I decided to go for it. The surgery wasn't bad, but the recovery was painful. It hurt to stand up, and I was on pain medication while I was recuperating. Getting used to the colostomy was weird at first. I felt like a baby because someone was always lifting my hospital gown to "burp" the bag. My bags now have a filter and burp themselves. (In 2016, my parents and I were at a restaurant when my colon let out a loud fart noise. Thankfully, nobody else heard it.)

Because it snowed while I was in the hospital, Mom and a nurse dressed me up to play outside and helped me build a miniature snowman. They let me take him inside to sit on my little table until he melted.

My cousin Kayla stayed with me during the day, and we tried to make the best of it. I can't thank her enough for everything. I wasn't coordinated and didn't want food in bed with me, so she fed me and did almost everything else.

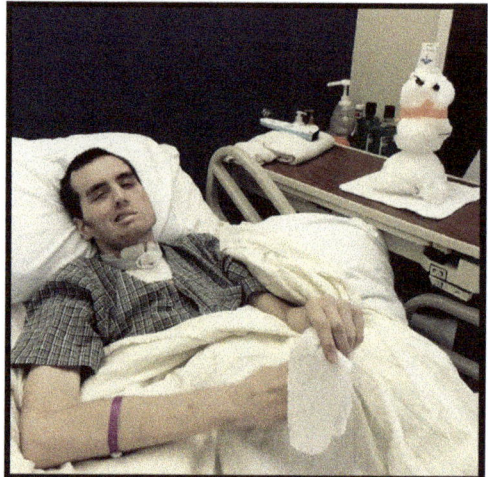

One day, Dad walked in the hospital room with Keybug, who was wearing a Nationals baseball hat. When Dad turned, I saw that he was wearing a jersey that had "Brown 20" on the back. Mom and Dad said Desi had bought those for me, so I texted him thank you and attached a picture of me holding the jersey. He texted back, "You can't get more authentic than that, straight from the club-house."

He later texted me a picture of his son wearing the Clemson shirt we bought. "We've got another Clemson fan!" he texted.

A few days later, a special bed arrived, and that meant one thing: I was going home! I was so excited that I sang "Home" by Daughtry in my head.

The drive home seemed to take forever. I hadn't seen my house in six long months—so long I hard-ly recognized it. When EMS opened the doors to get me out, I saw a redbrick building and thought it was a BBQ restaurant. *They must be hungry,* I thought. But my dad was smiling and saying, "Wel-come home, Ethan!"

Everything was great for a few weeks, and I was happy to be home. But I soon turned bitter toward everyone except my parents and Keybug. I was stuck in a hospital bed made especially for helping bedsores heal. All day, every day, I was in that bed, wishing my life were different. It was so boring that I actually looked forward to going to the wound care doctor weekly.

Since we had no means of transportation that wasn't painful for me, EMS sometimes came into the house and put me on the stretcher. Other times, Mom and Kayla would get me dressed and have me sit in my wheelchair in the garage until EMS came. When it got hotter, it was miserable in the ambulance because there was no air-conditioning.

My aunt Kelley and cousin Kristen would often come to the house unexpected, and I'd act angry, yell, or ignore them. If they tried to talk to me, which they always did, it was awkward because they didn't know much sign language. I look back at those times and feel very sad.

One night, an elderly couple came over along with my cousin Kristen and her mom. When Kristen tried to help my mom maneuver me, I wouldn't let her.

Her mom asked me, "Why are you so mean to us, especially my daughter?"

I was taken aback and angrily shouted that I wasn't.

My parents said, "You can be mean to us because we are your parents and will never leave, but you can't be mean to other people."

I told them that this wasn't easy for me. I'd lost my balance, my hearing, most of my vision, and the ability to speak clearly.

Being mean was just a mask I was hiding behind. I really wasn't angry with the people in my life but with the situation I was in. The people just happened to be the ones I took my anger out on, and I regret it now because that's not who I wanted to be.

Eventually, I remembered that every day we have a choice we have to make. We can be positive or negative. That's when I chose to be more positive.

* * *

As Mother's Day approached, my parents searched for a specially equipped van at a reasonable price. One day, I received a group text from our friend Sam Kelly:

Jan and Rick, I have been up for several hours now thinking about all of you—and the last several days too. Your Mother's Day gift from my family is a van for Ethan and all of you. I would like for you to go over to Carolina Mobility and pick out the van that you guys want and also pick out additional items and the easiest strapping down device they have. If they don't have the wheelchair accessible van you want in Greenville, they may have it at one of their other locations. We love you all very much. This is done and made possible because of Him, Jesus Christ our Lord. Happy Mother's Day to ALL of you!

Mom responded:

Oh, my goodness! Rick and I are absolutely just blown away by your generosity and love you have for us. We both have been crying because a weight has been lifted. Ethan asked me last night about going somewhere for his birthday, so I had to tell him we would just have to see how his wound was by then to get him in the car. Brad Jones also called yesterday and wanted Ethan to come to a fishing tournament at the end of the month. Now we can take him to meet the folks there. Ethan will be so excited to get out of the house. God has truly blessed us beyond measure! Thank you so very much! God bless you all!

I can't thank Sam enough for his friendship. He was there through my whole NF journey and one of the best friends I could've asked for. He also helped arrange a visit from C. J. Spiller by talking to the strength coach of the Buffalo Bills, Coach Ciano, who was recently named the best strength coach in the NFL.

After my wound started healing, I moved from sponge baths to actual baths. That terrified me because I had to keep a dry washcloth over the hole in my neck to keep from drowning, and that feeling didn't go away once the summer hit.

My family really enjoys the lake, and the ODF had weekly fishing trips. I asked my dad what would happen if the boat started to sink. How would I keep from drowning? He told me he'd keep my neck above water, but that didn't make me feel any better.

The problem was eventually solved one night in early January 2016 when my tube came out of my neck as I was sleeping, and the hole started to close.

The tube wouldn't fit in my neck properly, so Mom took me to the ER when she got off work.

My doctor was there, so he delivered the news himself: I could have it removed for good!

The feeding tube was a blessing and a curse. For the longest time, I had this plastic tube sticking out of my stomach that would often get pulled when I changed shirts. I tried to make the best of it. I took my medicine through it, and Keybug always wanted to help. He earned the name Doctor Keybug from Dad.

I eventually had that tube removed too, and I couldn't have been happier!

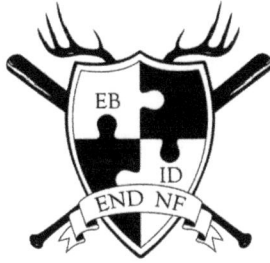

CHAPTER 12

Your attitude affects everything you do and has more impact than you think—not only on you, but also on others. During 2015, I felt a lot of anger and resentment. I had spent months in the hospital, had several surgeries, experienced almost constant pain from the bedsore, and wasn't recuperating nearly as well as I had expected.

I was at home in a hospital bed on total bed rest when I decided to text a friend who I'd known a long time. It started out with the usual, "How are you?" I was comfortable with her, so I opened up to her and told her what really was going on with me: I couldn't hear, my speech was slurred, my eyesight was terrible, and I would most likely never walk again.

I guess that was just too much for her to handle, so all she said was to "eat carrots, keep working hard, and I would get there."

I got defensive. We tried talking more, but I could sense something was wrong. When I asked what was bothering her, she answered, "You're being a total jerk! I was just trying to encourage you."

She was right. I really struggled with my attitude. In 2014, my dad asked my rehab doctor if he thought I'd walk again. The doctor said no. When Dad told me the news, I tried even harder in my sessions, but I never improved the way the staff wanted so I could appeal to the insurance company to allow me more sessions. When the doctor ordered more therapy in 2015, I figured that it was pointless. After a few more weeks of therapy without improvement, they discharged me. The truth was that I wasn't really trying. Sure, I wanted to walk again, but my attitude was bad. Why try if there was no hope?

But my parents kept trying. They urged me into therapy again, and I decided to change my attitude. You know what? I started seeing the results. I am still in my wheelchair, but I have tried to walk multiple times with weeks of physical therapy. Even though

I haven't improved like I wanted, that's okay. I just keep trying.

All I ask of others is that they keep trying. Why shouldn't I take my own advice? I may never walk again, but nobody will be able to say it's because I didn't keep trying.

There was a time when I let other people and social media control my mindset. I used to follow a good many NF Facebook pages, but I found that some people on the pages left depressing posts or comments, so I unfollowed them.

Actually, I was living a double life through social media. Facebook friends usually saw the positive, inspiring Ethan, but my Twitter followers saw a negative, uninspiring side of me. I lost a few followers by letting my negativity show, but it felt good to have a place to let it all out and to speak my mind. Not a lot of people use Twitter, so that was the place I put my true feelings.

The Facebook posts were a mask. People often said things like, "You're the strongest person I know," or "You're my hero." In all honesty, I may seem to have it all together. But my parents, Desi, and a few others know the truth. I have my bad days just like everyone.

Today, do I want to put on the strong, courageous, happy, heroic mask? Or do I show the real Ethan?

While it's good to be strong, courageous, happy, and heroic, a mask can be draining, both physically and mentally. Especially if it's all for show. I challenge you to put the real you on. It may be hard, but it won't be as draining as it would be if it's just for show.

My physical therapist once told me that I was too hard on myself. But I want to be driven; I'm a determined person. Always be you. Nobody can do it better.

In January 2019, our church voted in a new pastor. Mom and I met him at a meet and greet at church. He is an Alabama football fan, and after the beating Clemson gave them in the National Championship, I love to give him a hard time.

In one of his sermons, he said:

> I met a young man a few months ago that loves to give me a hard time. He says I'm a good pastor, but I pick terrible sport teams. That young man has touched my life in ways he will never understand. He told me one day that with all the suffering he goes through, he just wants to be used as a Christian who

*can point people to Jesus. I don't even need
to say his name because everyone knows who
I am referring to.*

He emails sermons to me and recently started putting Roll Tide (the rallying cry of Alabama) in the emails. Pastor, James 3:10 says, "Out of the same mouth come praise and cursing. My brothers and sisters, this should not be."

In November 2019, I posted a couple of videos to Facebook from physical therapy, showing me working on balance and lifting weights. Former Clemson football player Brandon Maye commented to say he's a fan.

You speak even when you don't realize it. Being faithful and determined in my therapy, with a good attitude, says a lot more than my words do.

For a long time, I prayed for a friend who wasn't family because family should always love you and stick with you no matter what. I wanted a friend who would do that. It took

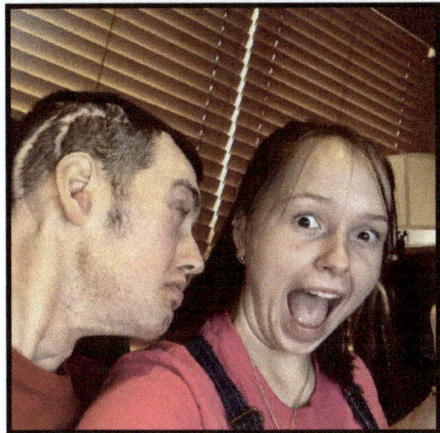

four years of praying and waiting before God finally brought me that friend.

First, I met her mom, Sheri, in 2015. She was my home nurse while I was recovering from the bedsore. Sheri was an excellent nurse and made sure I was comfortable during that painful time. While Sheri was my nurse, I met her daughters. One day, Amy, the older daughter, and I were going to watch a movie, and she asked if her younger sister Davida who was "kind of shy" could come too. Since I'm deaf, I asked Amy for Davida's number so I could invite her myself and make sure she wouldn't feel like just a tagalong.

Davida started texting me almost every day. After seeing how persistent she was—and more praying—I decided to give her a chance at the friendship she seemed to want.

People often tell me that they wished they had the time to learn sign language or to spend more time with me to understand my diagnosis. Davida is one of the busiest

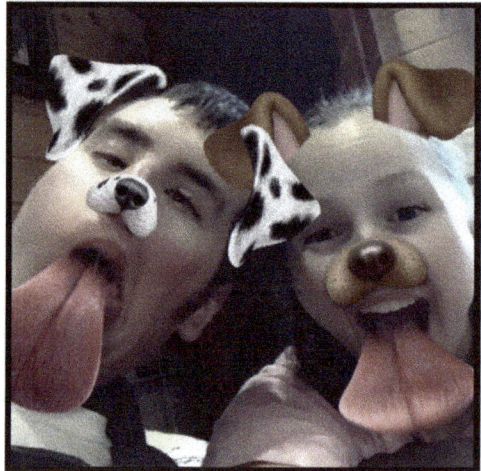

people I know. She has farm animals to take care of, including two baby goats and a dog, along with other responsibilities. Yet she finds time for me.

You do have the time. You make the time for what you really want to do. Davida immediately started learning sign language so that when I'm around her, I don't have to text her what I want to say and can quickly express myself. Her name is Sweet D in sign language. She is one of a few people who wanted to learn sign language so we could communicate. That, alone, shows how special she is.

She makes deaf jokes all the time just to make me laugh—but is quick to say *sorry* if she thinks she has offended me. There's a big difference in our ages, but we laugh and joke a lot. She's a little over five feet tall. During her freshman year of high school, she got to leave school early and excitedly told me she had a short day. I told her that every day is her short day.

Before Davida became my friend, I often struggled to get out of bed. When I woke up, I thought, *"It's just another day."* I usually dreaded it. When I went to therapy, I sometimes became ill and had to carry a vomit pan with me. Nerves, I guess. I'm usually pretty good at motivating myself, but sometimes Davida has to give me an extra little push to keep me going.

It's often said that the grass is greener on the other side of the fence. No, the grass is greener where you take the time to water it. Our driveway, like most, has grass on each side. Years ago, my dad bought some sod because it was cheap. It was brown, almost dead, and nobody wanted it. During the summer, since we often have droughts, he had me water it. I honestly didn't like doing it because it took my time and effort away from other things I wanted to do. But now that grass is as green, or greener, than the grass on the other side because we took the time to water it.

Sweet D sowed and watered a friendship with me. Now we're both reaping the benefits, and despite the age difference, we're best friends!

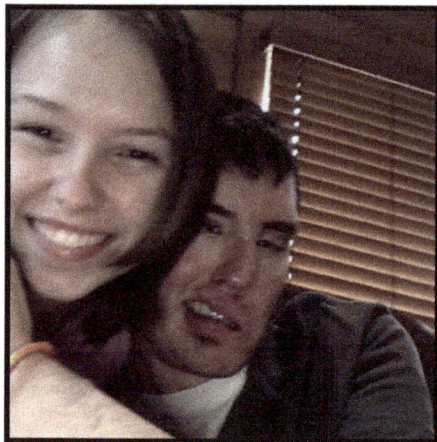

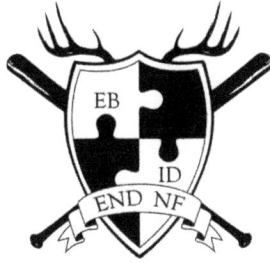

CHAPTER 13

In 2016, Keybug's mom told my mom that he could play baseball that year. I told Mom I would like to pay for him to play. At four years old, Keybug was "probably one of the best three (players) out there," according to the team evaluation to determine his skill set.

Keybug had not forgotten meeting Desi that first time. His T-ball coach asked him if he had played before. His response was that he had played with Ian Desmond!

Some time that year, my dad showed Keybug how to play video games on my Xbox. Friday through Sunday, I'd be in front of the TV playing games with him. Something that should take an hour to complete takes longer because he pauses the game and walks off or restarts it because he's losing.

I can't text when we play because he slaps my legs to get my attention.

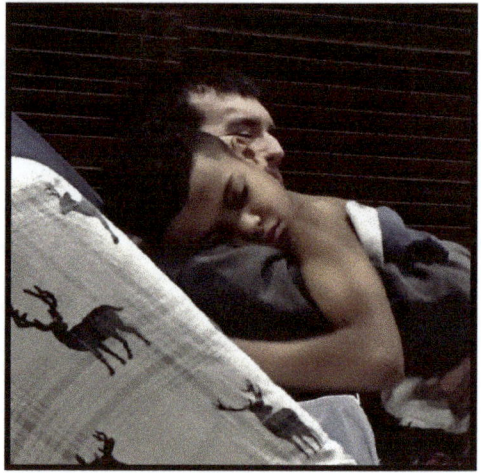

Of course, by this time, I'd already lost my hearing and, for the most part, my speech. But Keybug was too young to understand all my NF problems. As such, he has provided a couple of laughs. One Saturday, I was relaxing when Keybug asked me to play Xbox. I said, "Wait." Next thing I knew, I received a text from Mom saying, "Keybug told your dad and me, 'Ethan said his first word. Wait.'" He was so excited.

One day, Mom and I were hanging around while Keybug had team pictures taken. Mom said that a kid pointed at me and asked who I was. Keybug proudly said, "That's my brother!" I'm far from the brother he deserves, but he loves me anyway.

Keybug had a scrimmage after the pictures, so we went over to see him play. Keybug fielded the ball and went to tag the runner out at first base. When the two arrived at the base, he tackled the kid instead.

We signed him up for baseball but got football that day!

In 2017 and 2018, Keybug played again, and I'm happy to report that he didn't tackle anyone.

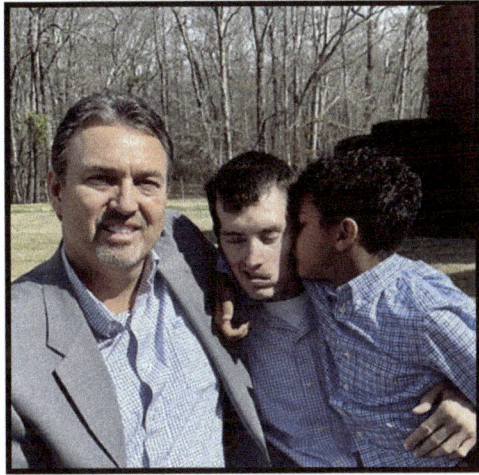

The 2019 baseball season was great for Keybug. Not only did he play well, but he did so well that he was selected to the eight-and-under All-Star Team while rocking Desi's Number 20 on his uniform.

Before we found out that he was selected to the All-Stars, we went to Atlanta. Desi texted Dad that he wanted to meet at Mizuno, a sporting goods store, where he treated Keybug to a signed bat, batting gloves, cleats, and a personalized fielding glove with "Keylen Rice #20" on it.

Our family, mainly my parents, were interviewed by the Rockies' TV crew, and I noticed Keybug taking it all in. I signed to Dad that Keybug was dreaming of playing there.

Growing up, I heard a song about making your life what you want it to be. Do your absolute best and don't stop until you reach your goal. If Keybug learns just one thing from me, I hope it's to always do his best and never give up. He's brought so much joy to my life and deserves nothing but the best.

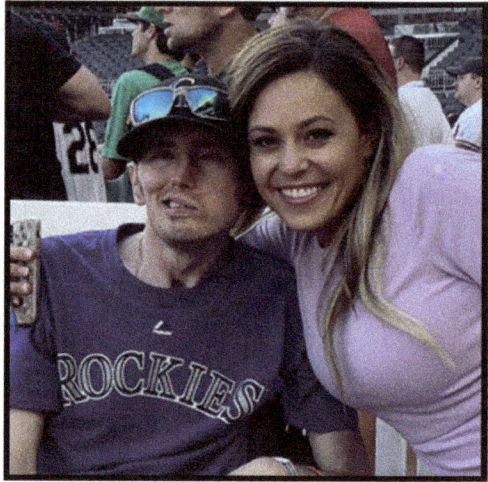

When I first started messaging Ian Desmond, Desi said that we might be able to learn from each other. Boy, has that ever been true. We've talked about everything from baseball to faith to NF. I will never forget those first direct messages on Twitter. They were the beginning of a relationship that I'll always cherish. That tweet to a stranger turned into text messages and telephone calls to a friend.

After getting his number, I would send him jokes or funny images because I knew it had to be tough being away from his family for days at a time. He had told me I could text him whenever I wanted, but I held back when he wasn't on road trips and during the off-season because I didn't want to take time from his family. When I told him that, he said,

"You're just like family."

I had always wanted a brother, but my parents couldn't have any more kids. Desi is the big brother I never had. We tease each other how I imagine blood brothers would. Desi usually used a blonde bat, but for one game, he used a black one. I asked what made him change.

"I switch it up some," he said. "Does the blonde look better on me?"

"I think it makes you look fat," I replied, "but that's just my opinion."

In 2014, we sealed our brotherhood forever by getting the matching tattoos promoting NF awareness.

To date, Desi has donated more than $75,000 to the Children's Tumor Foundation (CTF). The money is important as we work to end NF, but what's really important is that Desi gives his time to the families and kids affected by the disease. People wouldn't believe how many encouraging posts I have seen about him.

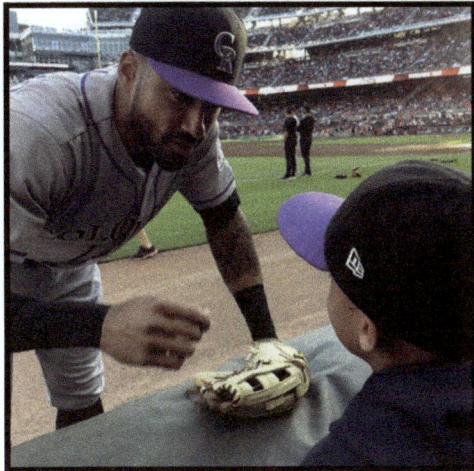

In a video interview with CTF, Desi said that he talks to me more than anyone else and that he feels the pain and emotions I feel. He is giving our fight to end NF a voice when we really didn't have one before him.

When I think of Desi and his impact on me and my family, I think of the song "Lean on Me" by Bill Withers. I can hear it in my head, and the words speak to me, reminding me that as we go through life, we all face pain, sorrow, and difficult times. In those times, I feel especially blessed to have someone like Desi, my brother, to lean on.

"As iron sharpens iron, so one person sharpens another" (Prov. 27:17).

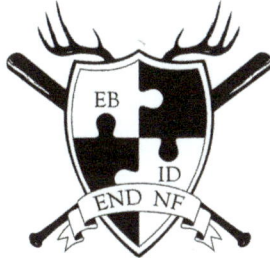

CHAPTER 14

If my mom has taught me anything, it's patience. My dad instructs me a lot. As I was growing up, he'd call it constructive criticism. I would tell him it was de-constructive and go to Mom. I'm a mama's boy, what can I say?

My parents' world turned upside down that summer in 2008, the year the radiologist told us I had brain tumors. They were devastated. Dad never gave up on trying to find the right doctor and treatment, and he found a doctor who traveled all over the world performing

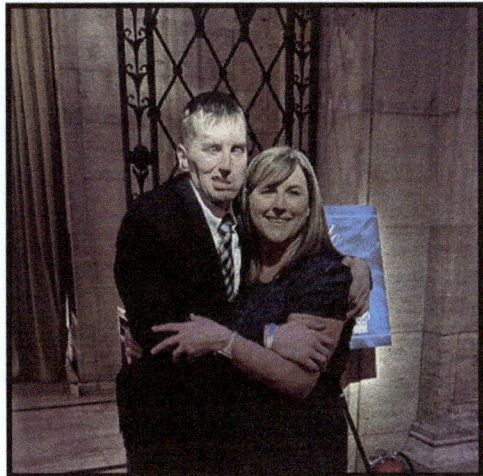

skull-based tumor surgery. He also did surgeries at Duke University in North Carolina.

My dad would walk through fire for me. "Listen, my son, to your father's instruction and do not forsake your mother's teaching" (Prov. 1:8).

My parents each wanted to include their perspective in this book. Here is a message from Mom:

> *Through it all, Ethan has kept his faith and been strong and courageous; a faithful friend; a wonderful son, grandson, nephew, and cousin; an inspiration; a light in a dark world. He has never lost his sense of humor, and he is my hero!*
>
> *Ethan does have bad days and gets down, but I tell him that it's okay to cry tonight, but joy comes in the morning. It's a new day to continue the fight.*
>
> *God always sends someone or something to encourage him. We've been so blessed to meet so many people we would have never known had we not been on this journey. I thank God every day for all their prayers and encouragement. God always gives us what we need when we need it!*

Here is a message from Dad:

As a parent, it was tough to see my son go through so many surgeries and so much suffering, missing out on a lot of things a normal teenager should be doing. But Ethan's faith was so strong, and even though he was having so many problems, he still reached out to help others. I admire his courage and faith through all this. I am not sure whether I could handle it the way he has. I am truly grateful for all the people who have come into our lives and made this journey more bearable.

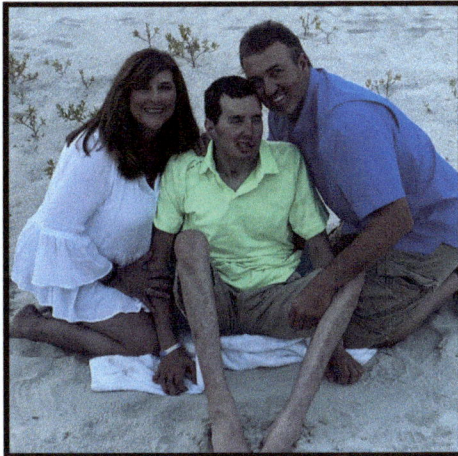

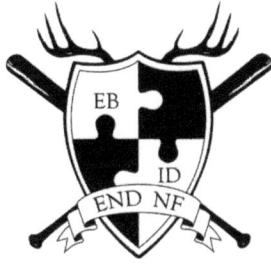

CHAPTER 15

On a public Facebook post once, I commented that even though I have this terrible disease called neurofibromatosis, God has been very good to me. Someone, an atheist, messaged me back, saying, "God's been good to you? You have this 'awful disease' and he can heal you but won't."

I believe to answer that question and others like it, we need to start with ourselves. In Genesis, God tells us He "created mankind in his own image, in the image of God he created them; male and female he created them" (Gen. 1:27). Not long after man's creation, along came a snake, embodied by Satan. We all know what happened right after that: trouble!

The evil serpent tempted Eve and made her question God. It asked her, "Did God really say you would die?" It was a question that begged for an answer and planted doubt in Eve's mind. The snake had her where he wanted her. Convinced that God was depriving her of something good, she ate of the forbidden fruit and then gave it to her husband, Adam. When God came to them later, he confronted them:

> *To the woman he said, "I will make your pains in childbearing very severe; with painful labor you will give birth to children. Your desire will be for your husband, and he will rule over you."*
>
> —Gen. 3:16

> *To Adam he said, "Because you listened to your wife and ate fruit from the tree about which I commanded you, 'You must not eat from it,' cursed is the ground because of you; through painful toil you will eat food from it all the days of your life. It will produce thorns and thistles for you, and you will eat the plants of the field. By the sweat of your brow you will eat your food until you return to the ground, since from it you were taken; for dust you are and to dust you will return."*
>
> —Genesis 3:17–19

As a Christian, I believe that God is all-good, all-loving, all-powerful, all-present, and all-knowing. You might ask, "If that's the case, then why did God allow Adam and Eve to sin? Or, if He knew they would sin, why didn't He intervene before it happened?"

Because of free will. When God made us, He made us with free will. You may think the punishment was severe for just eating fruit, but when the Bible says we were made in the image of God, it means that we were given morals. So, yes, Adam and Eve knew right from wrong, but the serpent got Eve to think that maybe God was holding out on them. If God had intervened, it would have reduced Adam and Eve to puppets. They probably wouldn't have sinned, but they couldn't have been fully free-willed.

If God is all-wise, then surely, He has good reasons for all the suffering. Think of the story of Job. Job knew all about pain and suffering. The beginning of the book of Job describes him as blameless and upright: "He feared God and shunned evil" (Job 1:1).

God asked Satan whether he'd considered Job and noticed that there were none like him in all the earth. Satan then claimed that Job loved God only because God had protected and blessed him so much. God and Satan made an agreement that allowed Satan to test Job with all kinds of suffering—anything short of killing him. Satan took all Job's earthly possessions, his home, and all ten of his children. Then he took his health. Through it all, Job didn't lose his integrity.

I can't begin to imagine the pain Job felt. I had a bedsore for a year, and it was some of the worst pain I ever felt. I lived on pain medicine in a special hospital bed specifically made to help bedsores heal. I spent all my time in that bed wishing I could play with Keybug. It was so tough for me as I watched Keybug grow closer to Dad because Dad could actually play with him. I taught him to like baseball, so I felt like it should be me helping him . . . not Dad.

Job's wife told him to curse God and die (Job 2:9–10), but he refused. The word for *integrity* can be translated into *innocence*. And here's the kicker: God didn't do any of this. It was all Satan's doing, though God did permit it.

When Job's friends heard about his suffering, they visited him and shared their thoughts on why he was suffering. His friends tried to comfort him with words, but all he really needed was their presence.

That's probably one reason there's a chair in a hospital room. During some of my hospitalizations, I wasn't able to speak to my visitors. But just knowing they cared enough to show up and sit with me was enough.

After his friends gave their answers, Job was filled with God's presence. Instead of answering all Job's questions, God asked one Himself: "Where were you when I laid the earth's foundation? Tell me, if you understand" (Job 38:4).

Recently, I was talking to my friend Hunter, who knew me before I was in a wheelchair, deaf, unable to talk clearly, drooling, and nearly blind. She said, "I don't understand why [bad stuff] happens to such amazing people." I thought, "*There are no good people.*" Yeah, I might be "good" in my eyes or in the eyes of other people. I've never committed a crime and have only been given a ticket for speeding. I've yelled at my parents out of frustration. I was sometimes rebellious and did things I shouldn't have done, but what kid hasn't? But how "good" is good enough? When we look at the Ultimate Good, God, we see that nobody measures up "for all have sinned and fall short of the glory of God" (Romans 3:23).

Growing up, I would often ask other people if they were Christians. Some would say, "No, but you don't have to be a Christian to be good."

I'd think, *"No, but I didn't ask if you were good. I asked if you were a Christian."* Being good isn't the issue. Isaiah 64:6 says that all our righteousness is like filthy rags in God's eyes because we are all sinners, bearing an inherited sin nature from Adam and Eve.

So, the issue is not that I was so good that I shouldn't have to suffer. I am a sinner, saved by grace. The issue to most people is why God allows anyone to suffer. At 16, I asked God, "Why me? What did I do to deserve this?" God used my mom, Ma-Ma, and a song by Building 429 called "You Carried Me" to help me understand.

Mom would tell me that I had to fight like Ma-Ma. "God didn't bring you this far to abandon you," she would say. The song still reminds me that—

> I stand only because you've given me grace to walk
> Only because
> You carried me
> You carried me through it all.[5]

---

5. Building 429, "You Carried Me" *Iris to Iris* (World Records, 2007), https://www.youtube.com/watch?v=64XDvdBqQ-o.

Do you think that if I had been given answers in those terrible times, they would've satisfied me? Absolutely not! I'd come back with more questions. The apostle Paul had what he called "a thorn in the flesh." He asked the Lord three times to be healed, but the Lord said, "My grace is sufficient for you, for my power is made perfect in weakness" (2 Cor. 12:9).

Through the years, I have seen how something that was devastating news to me has been used for good—even though some times were very hard. Since I was committed to lifting weights before my diagnosis, I worked hard and studied fitness magazines. But that past became a struggle for me once I could no longer lift. It wasn't the pictures in the magazines that made me hate who I was, but the pictures of my former self. I'd look at them and see a full smile; then I'd look at the pictures of me post-surgeries—with my half smile and stitched eyes—and get depressed.

It was draining to fake a smile and act like I was okay when I really wasn't. In 2013, at the rehabilitation hospital, I saw a psychologist and told her I just wanted to be *normal*.

She said, "That means *average*. You don't want to be average."

I wasn't placed here to be average.

There's an episode of *SpongeBob SquarePants* in which he thinks he's ugly, but in reality, he just has bad breath. His friend Patrick experiences the same problems, leading him to tell SpongeBob that he gave him "the ugly." I joke with Dad that he gave me the ugly. He teases back, "Your mom did."

I decided to accept who I am and make the best of my situation.

When I was 16 and going through my diagnosis and surgeries, my positivity influenced others positively. People I didn't know wrote to tell me, "Thank you." They'd tell me that their family started going back to church or that their life was different because of my story.

After Desi and I met, he told a media outlet that I encouraged and inspired him. When I thanked him for everything he has done for people with NF and the CTF organization, he said, "Dude, thank you! If it weren't for seeing your tweet, I wouldn't know about NF. Thank you for making me aware of it."

In 2015, my parents, my cousin Kayla, and I went to Atlanta to see Desi play. During batting practice, we were talking to him when one of his teammates, Dan Uggla, the second baseman, came over to us. He shook my hand and said he wanted to meet me because "Desi talks about you all the time."

In 2016, when Desi was playing for the Texas Rangers, a woman I didn't know tweeted me, saying, "Everybody in Texas knows your name."

In late 2017, I exchanged phone numbers with a guy named Tyler from Pennsylvania—a guy who knew me from Twitter after Desi gave me a "shout out." Tyler tweeted a picture of a wristband from the Children's Tumor Foundation and later told me that my story had a big impact on his life.

How can a guy from a small town in South Carolina—a guy who can't hear, speak clearly, or walk—influence people all over the country? I believe it all happened because God took my NF and used it for His glory.

You have to decide whether you will control your attitude about the things in your life or let them control you. C. S. Lewis said it best: "We regard God as an airman regards his parachute. It's there for emergencies but he hopes he never has to use it. . . . The real problem is not why some pious, humble, believing people suffer, but why some do not."[6]

Everything happened to me just as it was supposed to; believing that takes faith.[7]

---

6. C. S. Lewis, *The Problem of Pain* (New York: HarperCollins, 2001), 94–95.
7. For more reading on this topic, check out *The Problem of Pain* by C. S. Lewis and *How Could a Loving God* by Ken Ham.

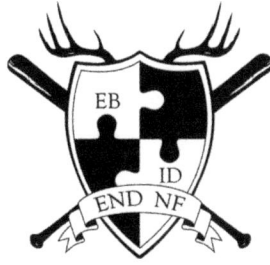

CHAPTER 16

When you're at your worst and it seems as though nobody wants or loves you, look to Jesus. He wants a relationship with you so much that He willingly died for you. If I look at myself, my situation, or my circumstances, I get depressed and fearful. But if I look at Jesus, I have peace. Worrying doesn't improve things; it can actually make them worse: "Can any one of you by worrying add a single hour to your life" (Matt. 6:27)?

But how do we turn to Jesus? Are you longing for Him as the deer longs for water (Ps. 42:1)? If so, good news! Jesus is the water of our salvation (John 4:14). In the New Testament book of Romans, a letter to the early Church in Rome, Paul outlines a simple path to salvation, sometimes called the

Romans Road. I invite you to come along as I walk down the Romans Road to salvation.

As I stated before, there are no good people. Don't just take my word for it. Romans 3:10 says, "As it is written: 'There is no one righteous, not even one.'" Romans 3:12 says, "All have turned away, they have together become worthless; there is no one who does good, not even one." Romans 5:12 says, "Therefore, just as sin entered the world through one man, and death through sin, and in this way death came to all people, because all sinned." This verse refers to Adam and Eve's sin, the original sin.

But is sin really that big of a deal? I know it's not popular in our society to think so, but yes, sin is a very big deal. Sin will take you farther than you want to go, cost you more than you want to pay, and keep you longer than you want to stay.

Sin is a big deal because "the wages of sin is death, but the gift of God is eternal life in Christ Jesus our Lord" (Rom. 6:23).

Salvation is God's free gift to us. We can't earn it by being good. "But God demonstrates his own love for us in this: While we were still sinners, Christ died for us" (Rom. 5:8).

You see, God loves us too much to leave us in this fallen state. After Adam and Eve sinned, God went looking for them. He promised them a Savior to restore them to Himself.

How can I be saved? "If you declare with your mouth, 'Jesus is Lord,' and believe in your heart that God raised him from the dead, you will be saved" (Rom. 10:9).

How can you be sure He heard you? "Everyone who calls on the name of the Lord will be saved" (Rom. 10:13).

In Matthew 14, Peter walked on water to meet Jesus, but when he looked around and feared the waves, he started to sink. He cried out to Jesus, "Lord, save me!" Jesus immediately reached for Peter and pulled him up. If you believe in Jesus and ask Him to save you today, He will do so immediately and forever.

When you're sealed in Jesus's love and redemption, you can experience the same peace I had the night before the surgery that made me completely deaf. "And the peace of God, which transcends all understanding, will guard your hearts and your minds in Christ Jesus" (Phil. 4:7).

The book of Romans says that God is the God of peace at least four times. By accepting Jesus, life won't necessarily be easier. In fact, it can be harder in some areas, and you may lose friends or even family. But I promise that He will be there with you to help you through.

Imagine standing before the Judge of heaven and earth. He looks at you with a stern look, reading the charges against you. "Son, you've lived a 'good' life by the world's standards, but you're a sinner, and sinners have no place in heaven. Take this sinner away from me!" says the Judge. As the handcuffs are slapped on, you hear a voice: "Father, I paid his debt on the cross!" The Judge looks at you and says, "Release him. He's forgiven!"

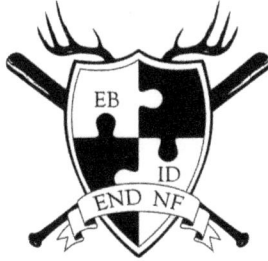

EPILOGUE

In November 2019, I had the opportunity to attend the Children's Tumor Foundation National 2019 Gala in New York City where Desi and I were honored and able to share the stage together. While there currently is no cure, efforts to end NF are underway. The gala raised $2.5 million toward those efforts.

The CTF also invited my parents and me to partner with them in their NF2 accelerator program, in which they expand the NF2 drug pipeline to get more treatments to clinics to help patients everywhere. I was thrilled to be involved. I learned in May 2020 that Desi is an honorary chairperson.

This book is another part of my activism. It was hard to revisit these memories and put them into words while enduring my ongoing health battles, but it was important for me to build awareness of this disease and continue the fight for a cure. If we don't have a voice, how can we be heard?

My prayer is that you'll continue educating yourself and get involved in NF awareness, join an NF walk, or a Cupid's Undie Run. Contact www.ctf.org for more information.

I'm hopeful every day that we'll find a cure. Until we do, I'll be fighting, praying, and spreading hope everywhere I can.

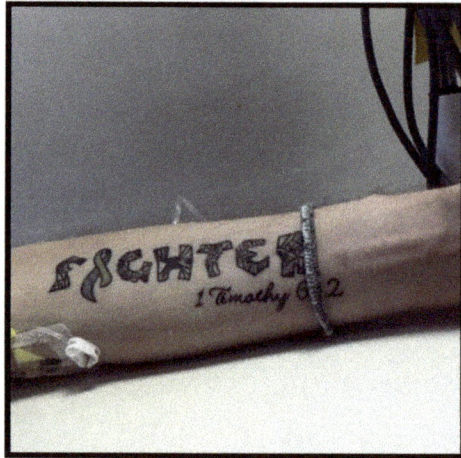

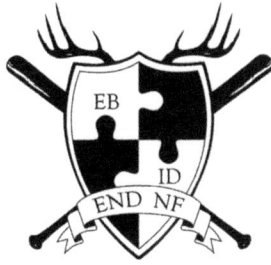

ACKNOWLEDGMENTS

I am skittish to do this page for fear I may miss people. It's hard to mention everyone in the "army," but here goes:

Thank you, Sam and Angie. Because of you, I am part of the awesome ODF and have a van that I love because I can go places. YBIC, Ethan.

Thank you, Four Fingers Frankie. As much as I want to see you in orange, please don't wear an orange speedo to this book signing. I cherish what vision I have.

Thank you, Dave and Brad Ruff, for each giving me your ODF auction items. I made some friends from what Brad gave me. Also, Rick Junior, enjoy this book and show me the money . . . all eight figures.

Thank you, Davida, for encouraging me throughout this. I can't count how many times you called this "the best book ever."

Thank you, Ann, for staying with me and always supporting this book.

Thank you, Michael, for being my first editor and encouraging me throughout this process. You helped me not to get discouraged.

Thank you, church family and family, for your prayers, support, and, most of all, love. I love you all. Thank you.

I would like to thank everyone who has encouraged me throughout the writing process, especially ODF members, including Mrs. Nancy, Dave, Freddy, and Wes.

A special thanks to my parents, particularly my mom, for standing by me through it all.

www.ingramcontent.com/pod-product-compliance
Lightning Source LLC
Chambersburg PA
CBHW040418110426
42813CB00013B/2696